Advancing Nuclear Medicine Through Innovation

Committee on State of the Science of Nuclear Medicine

Nuclear and Radiation Studies Board
Division of Earth and Life Studies

Board on Health Sciences Policy
Institute of Medicine

NATIONAL RESEARCH COUNCIL *AND*
INSTITUTE OF MEDICINE
OF THE NATIONAL ACADEMIES

THE NATIONAL ACADEMIES PRESS
Washington, D.C.
www.nap.edu

THE NATIONAL ACADEMIES PRESS 500 Fifth Street, N.W. Washington, DC 20001

NOTICE: The project that is the subject of this report was approved by the Governing Board of the National Research Council, whose members are drawn from the councils of the National Academy of Sciences, the National Academy of Engineering, and the Institute of Medicine. The members of the committee responsible for the report were chosen for their special competences and with regard for appropriate balance.

This study was supported by Contract No. DE-AM01-04PI45013, Task Order DE-AT01-06ER64218 between the National Academy of Sciences and the U.S. Department of Energy and Contract No. N01-OD-4-2139 between the National Academy of Sciences and the U.S. Department of Health and Human Services. Any opinions, findings, conclusions, or recommendations expressed in this publication are those of the author(s) and do not necessarily reflect the views of the organizations or agencies that provided support for the project.

International Standard Book Number-13: 978-0-309-11067-9 (Book)
International Standard Book Number-10: 0-309-11067-X (Book)
International Standard Book Number-13: 978-0-309-11068-6 (PDF)
International Standard Book Number-10: 0-309-11068-8 (PDF)

Additional copies of this report are available from the National Academies Press, 500 Fifth Street, N.W., Lockbox 285, Washington, DC 20055; (800) 624-6242 or (202) 334-3313 (in the Washington metropolitan area); Internet, http://www.nap.edu.

For more information about the Institute of Medicine, visit the IOM home page at: www.iom.edu.

Cover: Photo courtesy of Peter Conti, University of Southern California.

Printed in the United States of America.

THE NATIONAL ACADEMIES
Advisers to the Nation on Science, Engineering, and Medicine

The **National Academy of Sciences** is a private, nonprofit, self-perpetuating society of distinguished scholars engaged in scientific and engineering research, dedicated to the furtherance of science and technology and to their use for the general welfare. Upon the authority of the charter granted to it by the Congress in 1863, the Academy has a mandate that requires it to advise the federal government on scientific and technical matters. Dr. Ralph J. Cicerone is president of the National Academy of Sciences.

The **National Academy of Engineering** was established in 1964, under the charter of the National Academy of Sciences, as a parallel organization of outstanding engineers. It is autonomous in its administration and in the selection of its members, sharing with the National Academy of Sciences the responsibility for advising the federal government. The National Academy of Engineering also sponsors engineering programs aimed at meeting national needs, encourages education and research, and recognizes the superior achievements of engineers. Dr. Charles M. Vest is president of the National Academy of Engineering.

The **Institute of Medicine** was established in 1970 by the National Academy of Sciences to secure the services of eminent members of appropriate professions in the examination of policy matters pertaining to the health of the public. The Institute acts under the responsibility given to the National Academy of Sciences by its congressional charter to be an adviser to the federal government and, upon its own initiative, to identify issues of medical care, research, and education. Dr. Harvey V. Fineberg is president of the Institute of Medicine.

The **National Research Council** was organized by the National Academy of Sciences in 1916 to associate the broad community of science and technology with the Academy's purposes of furthering knowledge and advising the federal government. Functioning in accordance with general policies determined by the Academy, the Council has become the principal operating agency of both the National Academy of Sciences and the National Academy of Engineering in providing services to the government, the public, and the scientific and engineering communities. The Council is administered jointly by both Academies and the Institute of Medicine. Dr. Ralph J. Cicerone and Dr. Charles M. Vest are chair and vice chair, respectively, of the National Research Council.

www.national-academies.org

v

Reviewers

This report has been reviewed in draft form by individuals chosen for their diverse perspectives and technical expertise in accordance with procedures approved by the National Research Council's Report Review Committee. The purpose of this independent review is to provide candid and critical comments that will assist the institution in making its published report as sound as possible and to ensure that the report meets institutional standards of objectivity, evidence, and responsiveness to the study charge. The content of the review comments and draft manuscript remain confidential to protect the integrity of the deliberative process. We wish to thank the following individuals for their participation in the review of this report:

Simon Cherry, University of California, Davis
Chaitanya Divgi, University of Pennsylvania, Philadelphia
Ora Israel, Rambam Medical Center, Haifa, Israel
Jeanne Link, University of Washington, Seattle
Michael Phelps, University of California, Los Angeles
Theodore Phillips, University of California, San Francisco
Donald Podoloff, M.D. Anderson Cancer Center, Houston, Texas
Richard Reba, Georgetown University, Washington, D.C.
Kirby Vosburgh, Center for Integration of Medicine and Innovative
    Technologies, Cambridge, Massachusetts
Michael Welch, Washington University, St. Louis, Missouri

Chris Whipple, ENVIRON International Corporation, Emeryville, California
Paul Ziemer, Purdue University, West Lafayette, Indiana

Although the reviewers listed above have provided many constructive comments and suggestions, they were not asked to endorse the report's conclusions or recommendations, nor did they see the final draft of the report before its release. The review of this report was overseen by Floyd Bloom, Professor Emeritus, The Scripps Research Institute, and John Ahearne, Manager of the Ethics Program, Sigma Xi, The Scientific Research Society. Appointed by the National Research Council. They were responsible for making certain that an independent examination of this report was carried out in accordance with institutional procedures and that all review comments were carefully considered. Responsibility for the final content of this report rests entirely with the authoring committee and the National Research Council.

Preface

It has been an honor and a privilege to chair the committee on the state of science in nuclear medicine. As a diagnostic radiologist, a clinician-scientist, and the chairperson of a large academic radiology department, I have been exposed to the many advances in nuclear medicine and have observed their clinical benefits up close. Participating in this review, however, has allowed me to step back and appreciate the magnitude of the progress that has been achieved, and the crucial role that government funding has played in it. Investments in chemistry, physics, engineering, and training are responsible for the state-of-the-art radiopharmaceuticals and imaging instruments that we now rely on to improve our understanding of human physiology through non-invasive disease detection and treatment monitoring.

These advances have already had a major impact on all branches of imaging and medicine, yet, they pale in comparison to those on the horizon. Nuclear medicine offers a unique, non-invasive view into intracellular processes and enzyme trafficking, receptors and gene expression, and forms the theoretical and applied foundation for molecular medicine. The contributions of nuclear medicine are creating the possibility of a future of personalized medicine, in which treatments and medications will be based on an individual's unique genetic profile and response to disease processes.

Although the progress in nuclear medicine research in the United States has been spectacular, potential obstacles to its continuation have been noted in previous reports, including a critical shortage of chemists and other personnel trained in nuclear medicine, and an inadequate supply of radionuclides for research and development. In addition, uncertainty has arisen about how, and to what degree, the government should continue to fund nuclear medicine research. For years, the basic chemistry and physics research behind the growth of the field has been supported by the Medical Applications and Sciences Program of the Department of Energy (DOE) Office of Biological and Environmental Research. However, the uniqueness of this program relative to the nuclear medicine research funded by the National Institutes of Health (NIH) has long been under debate. The DOE and the NIH commissioned this study on the state of the science in nuclear medicine because of the uncertainty surrounding the support of the Medical Applications and Sciences Program. Specifically, the sponsoring agencies asked that the National Academies assess areas of need in nuclear medicine research, examine the program and make recommendations to improve its impact on nuclear medicine research and isotope production.

In response to this request, the National Research Council of the National Academies appointed a committee of 14 experts to carry out this study. The committee gathered information from members of the public, experts on nuclear medicine, scientific and medical societies, and federal agencies. In composing its report, the committee decided to describe the needs in nuclear medicine research primarily in terms of future opportunities in the field. Thus the report, in my view, is an exciting, forward-looking document that makes clear the potential of the field for further advancing medicine, and suggests practical steps to facilitate progress. I hope and believe that it will have a positive impact on the future of nuclear medicine.

Hedvig Hricak, *Chair*

Acknowledgments

The committee is grateful to the speakers and panelists (listed in Appendix A) who participated in the information-gathering sessions for the study. In addition, the committee wishes to thank Belinda Seto, Peter Preusch, and Dan Sullivan at the National Institutes of Health (NIH); and Mike Viola, John Pantaleo, Prem Srivastava, and Peter Kirschner at the Department of Energy (DOE) for contributing their time, efforts, and insights to the study.

I would like to personally thank my fellow committee members for their dedication to carrying out a thorough study and writing a useful report. They all cared deeply about the topic, and their probing questions and lively discussions ensured that we covered a wide range of issues and considered them from multiple angles.

Studies such as this are often long on information and short on time, and the committee would like to thank the many National Research Council staff members whose help was essential in producing this report. Among these, the committee particularly wishes to acknowledge Kevin Crowley, Director of the Nuclear and Radiation Studies Board, for providing guidance on the study process and keeping the committee focused on its charge; Shaunteé Whetstone and James Yates for their administrative support; Toni Greenleaf for making sure that we stayed on budget; and Rick Jostes for his technical contributions to the report. I would especially like to thank the

Study Director, Naoko Ishibe, for her devotion to the project, and particularly for her superb work in coordinating the writing of the report. Finally, I am grateful to the DOE and NIH for sponsoring this study.

Hedvig Hricak, *Chair*

Contents

SUMMARY   1

1   INTRODUCTION   10
    Strategy to Address the Study Charge, 14
    Report Roadmap, 15

2   NUCLEAR MEDICINE   17
    Significant Discoveries, 22
    Frontiers in Nuclear Medicine, 23
    Complexities of Nuclear Medicine Practice and Research, 38
    Conclusion, 42

3   NUCLEAR MEDICINE IMAGING IN DIAGNOSIS
    AND TREATMENT   43
    Background, 43
    Current State of Nuclear Medicine Imaging and Emerging
        Priorities, 44
    Impediments to Progress and Current and Future Needs, 56

4   TARGETED RADIONUCLIDE THERAPY   59
    Background, 60
    Significant Discoveries, 65
    Current State of the Field and Emerging Priorities, 66
    Current Impediments to Full Implementation of Targeted
        Radiopharmaceutical Therapeutics, 72

Recommendations, 73
Conclusions, 74

5   AVAILABILITY OF RADIONUCLIDES FOR NUCLEAR
    MEDICINE RESEARCH   75
    Background, 75
    Significant Discoveries, 76
    Current State of Radionuclide Availability in the United States, 80
    Current and Future Needs, 83
    Recommendations, 87

6   RADIOTRACER AND RADIOPHARMACEUTICAL
    CHEMISTRY   89
    Background, 89
    Significant Discoveries, 90
    Current State of the Field and Emerging Priorities, 93
    Current Needs and Impediments, 101
    Recommendations, 102

7   INSTRUMENTATION AND COMPUTATIONAL SCIENCES   104
    Background, 104
    Significant Discoveries, 107
    Current State of the Field and Emerging Priorities, 111
    Future Needs, 114
    Findings, 116
    Recommendations, 117

8   EDUCATION AND TRAINING OF NUCLEAR
    MEDICINE PERSONNEL   118
    Background, 118
    Current Status of the Workforce, 119
    Findings, 129
    Recommendations, 130

REFERENCES   131

APPENDIXES
A   INFORMATION-GATHERING SESSIONS   141
B   GLOSSARY AND ACRONYMS   146
C   COMMERCIALLY AVAILABLE RADIOPHARMACEUTICALS   151
D   BIOGRAPHICAL SKETCHES OF COMMITTEE MEMBERS   155

Summary

T he history of nuclear medicine over the past 50 years reflects the strong link between government investments in science and technology and advances in health care in the United States and worldwide. As a result of these investments, new nuclear medicine procedures have been developed that can diagnose diseases non-invasively, providing information that cannot be acquired with other imaging technologies; and deliver targeted treatments. Nearly 20 million nuclear medicine procedures using radiopharmaceuticals and imaging instruments are carried out annually in the United States alone. Overall usage of nuclear medicine procedures is expanding rapidly, especially as new imaging technologies, such as positron emission tomography/computed tomography (PET/CT) and single photon emission computed tomography/computed tomography (SPECT/CT), continue to improve the accuracy of detection, localization, and characterization of disease, and as automation and miniaturization of cyclotrons and advances in radiochemistry make production of radiotracers more practical and versatile.

Recent advances in the life sciences (e.g., molecular biology, genetics, and proteomics[1]) have stimulated development of better strategies for detecting and treating disease based on an individual's unique profile, an approach that is called "personalized medicine." The growth of personalized medicine will be aided by research that provides a better understanding of normal and pathological processes; greater knowledge of the mechanisms

---

[1]Proteomics is the study of the structure and function of proteins, including the way they interact with each other in cells.

by which individual diseases arise; superior identification of disease subtypes; and better prediction of an individual patient's responses to treatment. However, the process of advancing patient care is complex and slow. Expanded use of nuclear medicine techniques has the potential to accelerate, simplify, and reduce the costs of developing and delivering improved health care and could facilitate the implementation of personalized medicine.

Current clinical applications of nuclear medicine include the ability to:

- diagnose diseases such as cancer, neurological disorders (e.g., Alzheimer's and Parkinson's diseases), and cardiovascular disease in their initial stages, permitting earlier initiation of treatment as well as reduced morbidity and mortality;
- non-invasively assess therapeutic response, reducing patients' exposure to the toxicity of ineffective treatments and allowing alternative treatments to be started earlier; and
- provide molecularly targeted treatment of cancer and certain endocrine disorders (e.g., thyroid disease and neuroendocrine tumors).

Emerging opportunities in nuclear medicine include the ability to:

- understand the relationship between brain chemistry and behavior (e.g., addictive behavior, eating disorders, depression);
- assess the atherosclerotic cardiovascular system;
- understand the metabolism and pharmacology of new drugs;
- assess the efficacy of new drugs and other forms of treatments, speeding their introduction into clinical practice;
- employ targeted radionuclide therapeutics to individualize treatment for cancer patients by tailoring the properties of the targeting vehicle and the radionuclide;
- develop new technology platforms (e.g., integrated microfluidic chips and other automated screening technologies) that would accelerate and lower the cost of discovering and validating new molecular imaging probes, biomarkers, and radiotherapeutic agents;
- develop higher resolution, more sensitive imaging instruments to detect and quantify disease faster and more accurately;
- further develop and exploit hybrid imaging instruments, such as positron emission tomography/magnetic resonance imaging (PET/MRI), to improve disease diagnosis and treatment; and
- improve radionuclide production, chemistry, and automation to lower the cost and increase the availability of radiopharmaceuticals by inventing a new miniaturized particle accelerator and associated technologies

to produce short-lived radionuclides for local use in research and clinical programs.

In spite of these exciting possibilities, deteriorating infrastructure and loss of federal research support are jeopardizing the advancement of nuclear medicine. It is critical to revitalize the field to realize its potential.

CHARGE TO THE COMMITTEE

The National Academies were asked by the Department of Energy (DOE) and the National Institutes of Health (NIH) to review the state of the science of nuclear medicine in response to discussions between the DOE and the Office of Management and Budget about the future scientific areas of research for the DOE's Medical Applications and Sciences Program. In response to this request, the National Academies formed the Committee on the State of the Science of Nuclear Medicine. The committee's mandate was to review the current state of the science in nuclear medicine; identify future opportunities in nuclear medicine research; and identify ways to reduce the barriers that impede both basic and translational research (Sidebar 1.1). Although the committee is aware that funds will be required to implement the recommendations made in this report, providing funding recommendations is beyond the scope of the committee's charge. This report reflects the consensus views and judgments of the committee members, based in part on consultation with experts from academia, major medical societies, relevant governmental agencies, and industry representatives.

FINDINGS AND RECOMMENDATIONS

Advances on the horizon in nuclear medicine could substantially accelerate, simplify, and reduce the cost of delivering and improving health care. To realize this promise, we need to focus research on the following: (1) the development of new radionuclide production facilities and technologies; (2) the synthesis of new radiotracers to improve understanding of how specific organs function; (3) the development of imaging instruments, enabling technologies, and multimodality imaging devices, such as PET/CT and PET/MRI, to improve disease diagnosis; (4) the development and use of targeted radionuclide therapeutics that will allow cancer treatments to be tailored for individual patients; (5) the use of nuclear medicine imaging as a tool in the discovery and development of new drugs; and (6) the translation of research from bench to bedside, including investment in training of clinician scientists in nuclear medicine techniques. Specific research opportunities are discussed in Chapters 3, 4, 6, and 7 of the report. Achieving these research goals will require collaboration among academic institutions, industry, and federal agencies.

FINDING 1: Loss of Federal Commitment for Nuclear Medicine Research.

FINDING 1A: The Medical Applications and Sciences Program[2] under the DOE's Office of Biological and Environmental Research (DOE-OBER) (and precursor agencies, Atomic Energy Commission and Energy Research and Development Administration) has provided a platform for the conceptualization, discovery, development, and translation of basic science in chemistry and nuclear and particle physics for several decades (examples include FDG-PET,[3] technetium-99m SPECT, targeted radionuclide therapy). In fiscal year (FY) 2006, Congress reduced funding of the program by 85 percent (Figure S.1).

The committee finds that as a result of this reduction in funding, there

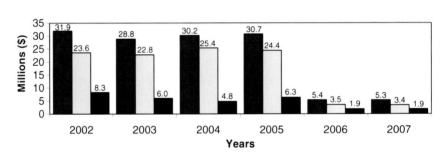

FIGURE S.1 DOE-OBER funding for nuclear medicine research, 2002—2007. SOURCE: DOE-OBER.

has been a substantial loss of support for the physical sciences and engineering basic to nuclear medicine. There is now no specific programmatic long-term commitment by any federal agency for maintaining high-technology infrastructure (e.g., accelerators, research reactors) or centers for instrumentation and chemistry research and training, which are at the heart of nuclear medicine research and development (Chapters 6 and 7).

---

[2]DOE-OBER Medical Applications and Measurement Sciences Program provided federal support for basic scientific studies in nuclear medicine.

[3]FDG is 2-deoxy-2-[18F]fluoro-D-glucose, also called fluorodeoxyglucose.

FINDING 1B: The DOE-Nuclear Energy (NE) Isotope Program is not meeting the needs of the research community because the effort is not adequately coordinated with NIH activities or with the DOE-OBER (Chapter 5).

FINDING 1C: Public Law 101-101, which requires full-cost recovery for DOE-supplied isotopes, whether for clinical use or research, has restricted research isotope production and radiopharmaceutical research. The lack of new commercially available radiotracers over the past decade may be due in part to this legislation (Chapter 5).

RECOMMENDATION 1: *Enhance the federal commitment to nuclear medicine research. Given the somewhat different orientations of the DOE and the NIH toward nuclear medicine research, the two agencies should find some cooperative mechanism to support radionuclide production and distribution; basic research in radionuclide production, nuclear imaging, radiopharmaceutical/radiotracer and therapy development; and the transfer of these technologies into routine clinical use (Chapter 6).*

    Implementation Action 1A: Reinstating support for the DOE-OBER nuclear medicine research program should be considered.

    Implementation Action 1B: A national nuclear medicine research program should be coordinated by the DOE and the NIH with the former emphasizing the general development of technology and the latter disease-specific applications. In committing itself to the stewardship of technology development (radiopharmaceuticals and imaging instrumentation), the DOE would reclaim a leadership role in this field.

    Implementation Action 1C: In developing their strategic plan, the agencies should avail themselves of advice from a broad range of authorities in academia, the national laboratories, and industry; these authorities should include experts in physics, engineering, computer science, chemistry, radiopharmaceutical science, commercial development, regulatory affairs, clinical trials, and radiation biology.

FINDING 2: Cumbersome Regulatory Requirements.

There are three primary impediments to the efficient entry of promising new radiopharmaceutical tracer compounds into clinical feasibility studies: (1) complex U.S. Food and Drug Administration (FDA) toxicologic and other regulatory requirements (i.e., lack of regulatory pathways specifically for both diagnostic and therapeutic radiopharmaceuticals that take into account the unique properties of these agents); (2) lack of specific guidelines from the FDA for good manufacturing practice for PET radiodiagnostics and other radiopharmaceuticals; and (3) lack of a consensus for standardized image acquisition in nuclear medicine imaging procedures and harmonization of protocols appropriate for multi-institutional clinical trials (Chapters 3, 4, and 6).

RECOMMENDATION 2: Clarify and simplify regulatory requirements, including those for (A) toxicology and (B) current good manufacturing practices (cGMP) facilities (Chapters 3 and 4).

Implementation Action 2A, Toxicology: The FDA should clarify and issue final guidelines for performing pre-investigational new drug evaluation for radiopharmaceuticals, particularly with regard to the recently added requirement for studies to determine late radiation effects for targeted radiotherapeutics.

Implementation Action 2B, cGMP: The FDA should issue final guidelines on cGMP for radiopharmaceuticals. These guidelines should be graded commensurate with the properties, applications, and potential risks of the radiopharmaceuticals, instead of regulating minimal-risk compounds with the same degree of stringency as de novo compounds and new drugs that have pharmacologic effects.

Implementation Action 2C: To develop prototypes of standardized imaging protocols for multi-institutional clinical trials, members of the imaging community should meet with representatives of federal agencies (e.g., DOE, NIH, FDA) to discuss standardization, validation, and pathways for establishing surrogate markers of clinical response.

FINDING 3: Inadequate Domestic Supply of Medical Radionuclides for Research.

There is no domestic source for most of the medical radionuclides used in day-to-day nuclear medicine practice. Furthermore, the lack of a dedicated domestic accelerator and reactor facilities for year-round uninterrupted production of medical radionuclides for research is discouraging the development and evaluation of new radiopharmaceuticals. The parasitic use[4] of high-energy physics machines has failed to meet the needs of the medical research community with regard to radionuclide type, quantity, timeliness of production, and affordability (Chapters 4, 5, and 6).

---

[4]Accelerators that have been made available for the production of radionuclides, although the machines are in operation for other purposes.

RECOMMENDATION 3: *Improve domestic medical radionuclide production. To alleviate the shortage of accelerator- and nuclear reactor-produced medical radionuclides available for research, a dedicated accelerator and an appropriate upgrade to an existing research nuclear reactor should be considered (Chapters 4 and 5).*

This recommendation is consistent with other studies that have reviewed medical radionuclide supply in the United States and have come to the same conclusions (IOM 1995, Wagner et al. 1999, Reba et al. 2000).

FINDING 4: Shortage of Trained Nuclear Medicine Scientists.

FINDING 4A: There is a critical shortage of clinical and research personnel in all nuclear medicine disciplines (chemists, radiopharmacists, physicists, engineers, clinician-scientists, and technologists) with an impending "generation gap" of leadership in the field. Training, particularly of radiopharmaceutical chemists, has not kept up with current demands at universities, medical institutions, and industry, a problem that is exacerbated by a shortage of university faculty in nuclear chemistry and radiochemistry (NRC 2007). There is a pressing need for additional training programs with the proper infrastructure to support interdisciplinary science, more doctoral students, and post-doctoral fellowship opportunities (Chapter 8).

RECOMMENDATION 4A: *Train nuclear medicine scientists. To address the shortage of nuclear medicine scientists, engineers, and research physicians, the NIH and the DOE, in conjunction with specialty societies, should consider convening expert panels to identify the most critical national needs for training and determine how best to develop appropriate curricula to train the next generation of scientists and provide for their support (Chapter 8).*

FINDING 4B: With the current decline in the number of U.S. students going into chemistry, the restriction of training grants to U.S. citizens and permanent residents as required by the Public Health Service Act is a substantial impediment to recruitment of new talent into the field (Chapter 8).

RECOMMENDATION 4B: *Provide additional, innovative training grants. To address the needs documented in this report, specialized instruction of chemists from overseas could be accomplished in some innovative fashion (particularly in DOE-supported programs) by linking training to research. This might take the form of subsidies for course development and delivery as well as tuition subventions. By directly linking training to specific re-*

search efforts, such subventions would differ from conventional NIH/DOE training grants (Chapter 8).

FINDING 5: Need for Technology Development and Transfer.

FINDING 5A: There is an urgent need for the further development of highly specific technology and of targeted radiopharmaceuticals for disease diagnosis and treatment. Improvements in detector technology, image reconstruction algorithms, and advanced data processing techniques, as well as development of lower cost radionuclide production technologies (e.g., a versatile, compact, short-lived radionuclide production source), are among the research areas that should be explored for effective translation into the clinic. Such technology development frequently needs long incubation periods and cannot be carried out in standard 3- to 5-year funding cycles (Chapters 6 and 7).

FINDING 5B: Transfer of technological discoveries from the laboratory to the clinic is critical for advancing nuclear medicine. Historically, federally funded research and development has driven the development of instrumentation and radiotracers that form the backbone of nuclear medicine practice worldwide. These discoveries have largely been due to the proximity of scientific disciplines in nuclear science and technology. Capitalizing on this multi-disciplinary mix has served nuclear medicine well in the past and could do so in the future (Chapter 7).

RECOMMENDATION 5: *Encourage interdisciplinary collaboration. The DOE-OBER should continue to encourage collaborations between basic chemistry, physics, computer science, and imaging laboratories, as well as multi-disciplinary centers focused on nuclear medicine technology development and application, to stimulate the flow of new ideas for the development and translation of next-generation radiopharmaceuticals and imaging instrumentation. The role of industry should be considered and mechanisms developed that would hasten the technology development process (Chapters 6 and 7).*

LOOKING AHEAD

Groundbreaking work in genomics, proteomics, and molecular biology is rapidly increasing our understanding of disease processes and disease management. As a result, we now have the opportunity to develop highly personalized medicine, in which each patient and disease can be individually characterized at the molecular level to identify the treatment strategies that will be most effective. Nuclear medicine techniques that image biochemical function in vivo can facilitate the development and implementation of such tailored treatment. However, while history highlights the payoff and public benefit from government investments in science and technology for nuclear medicine, the competitive edge that the United States has held for the past 50 years is seriously challenged. Three major impediments have been identified:

1.   There is no short- or long-term programmatic commitment by any agency to funding chemistry, physics, and engineering research and associated high-technology infrastructure (accelerators, instrumentation, and imaging physics), which are at the heart of nuclear medicine technology research and development.

2.   There is no domestic supplier for most of the radionuclides used in day to day nuclear medicine practice in the United States and no accelerator dedicated to research on medical radionuclides needed to advance targeted molecular therapy in the future.

3.   Training for nuclear medicine scientists, particularly for radiopharmaceutical chemists, has not kept up with current demands in universities and industry, a problem that is exacerbated by a shortage of university faculty in nuclear and radiochemistry.

Thus, although the scientific opportunities have never been greater or more exciting, the infrastructure on which future innovations in nuclear medicine depend hangs in the balance. If the promise of the field is to be fulfilled, a federally supported infrastructure for basic and translational research in nuclear medicine should be considered.

1

Introduction

This study was prompted by discussions between the U.S. Department of Energy (DOE) and the Office of Management and Budget (OMB) about future scientific areas for the DOE Office of Biological and Environmental Research Medical Applications and Sciences Program.[1] OMB recommended that program functions be retained, but that funds for the program be reduced beginning in fiscal year (FY) 2006. However, they agreed to delay decisions about program restructuring pending a state-of-the-science review of nuclear medicine from the National Academies. In FY 2006, Congress passed and the President signed an 85 percent ($23 million) reduction in the funding for the DOE budget for basic nuclear medicine and molecular imaging research, leaving only support for the neuroimaging program at Brookhaven National Laboratory[2, 3] (Figure 1.1).

Historically, basic nuclear medicine research has been funded primarily by the DOE and its predecessor agencies, the Atomic Energy Commission (AEC) and the Energy Research and Development Administration (ERDA) (DOE 2007a, DOE 2007b). The desire to apply radioactivity's promise for peaceful use instigated a transfer of research in atomic energy from the War Department to AEC in 1947. Its mission was to oversee research pro-

---

[1] DOE's Office of Biological and Environmental Research (DOE-OBER) Medical Applications and Measurement Sciences Program provides federal support for basic scientific studies in nuclear medicine.

[2] Joanna Fowler is the Director of the Center for Translational Neuroimaging at Brookhaven National Laboratory.

[3] An earmark appropriation continued a program at UCLA as well.

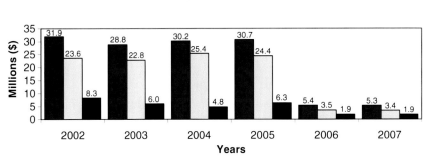

FIGURE 1.1 DOE-OBER funding for nuclear medicine research, 2002—2007.
SOURCE: Data provided by DOE-OBER.

grams in health measures and radiation biology conducted at the national
laboratories. Subsequently, the Energy Reorganization Act of 1974 created
ERDA, which assumed and expanded on AEC's responsibilities. Three years
later, the DOE was created. Within the DOE, the Office of Nuclear Energy
(DOE-NE) provides radionuclides to the research community on a full-cost-
recovery basis through its Isotope Program, while the DOE-OBER provides
federal support for basic scientific studies in nuclear medicine through its
Medical Applications and Measurement Sciences Program.

The mission of the program has been "to deliver relevant scientific
knowledge that will lead to innovative diagnostic and treatment technologies for human health." The specific objectives of the program are as follows (DOE 2006):

1. to utilize innovative radiochemistry to develop new radiotracers for
medical research, clinical diagnosis, and treatment;

2. to develop the next generation of non-invasive nuclear medicine
technologies;

3. to develop advanced imaging detection instrumentation capable of
high resolution from the sub-cellular to the clinical level; and

4. to utilize the unique resources of the DOE in engineering, physics,
chemistry, and computer sciences to develop the basic tools to be used in
biology and medicine, particularly in imaging sciences, photo-optics and
biosensors.

The program directly supported nuclear medicine research through
radiopharmaceutical and instrument development and the development of

radionuclides for diagnosis and targeted therapy (Chapter 4).[4] It also supported dedicated cyclotrons[5] for the production of short-lived, positron[6]-emitting radionuclides for use in NIH clinical research.

In FY 2005, the program provided approximately $30 million in federal research support for facilities and scientific investigations at seven national laboratories and 35 universities. Over the years, research supported by this program has provided new technological and clinical tools in nuclear medicine that have resulted in medical breakthroughs. For example, the research has enabled:

  • the development of positron emission tomography (PET) scanners to diagnose and monitor the treatment of cancer and other diseases;
  • the advancement of radiotracer chemistry, leading to the synthesis of fluorine-18-labeled fluorodeoxyglucose (FDG)[7] and many other tracers for imaging the human brain and other organs with PET;
  • the development of the molybdenum-99m/technetium-99m generator, which is the most widely used tracer in nuclear medicine, worldwide; and
  • further advances in the application of "exotic" therapeutic pharmaceuticals, such as the alpha-particle emitters that have great promise for cancer therapy.

Additional discoveries and developments are highlighted in Chapter 2.

Funding for nuclear medicine has also come from the National Institutes of Health (NIH), particularly the National Cancer Institute (NCI) and, more recently, the National Institute of Biomedical Imaging and Bioengineering (NIBIB). In FY 2006, $44.7 million and $17.8 million were expended by NCI and NIBIB, respectively, for extramural nuclear medicine research (Figure 1.2). Other Institutes,[8] such as the National Institute of Mental Health, have also funded nuclear medicine research ($70.8 million in FY 2006 for both intramural and extramural programs). However, an informal analysis of NIH's nuclear medicine portfolio suggests that ap-

---

[4]Targeted radionuclide therapy is a form of treatment that delivers therapeutic doses of radiation to malignant tumors, for example, by administration of a radiolabeled molecule into the blood stream that is designed to seek out certain cells.

[5]A cyclotron (Sidebar 5.1) is a machine used to accelerate charged particles to high energies.

[6]A positron is an elementary particle of antimatter that undergoes mutual annihilation with a nearby electron, which produces two gamma rays traveling in the opposite direction.

[7]The use of FDG with PET scan technology has now been validated and its importance documented in the diagnosis, staging, and follow-up of approximately two dozen different types of malignancies.

[8]Data were not available for the National Heart, Lung, and Blood Institute, the National Institute of Neurological Disorders and Stroke, and the National Institute of Drug Abuse.

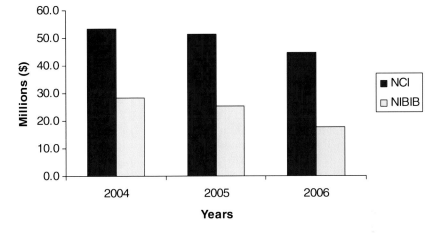

FIGURE 1.2 Extramural funding for nuclear medicine research, 2004—2006. SOURCE: Data provided by NCI and NIBIB.

proximately 75 percent of these funds represent *application* of currently available radiotracers and technologies (e.g., FDG-PET) rather than fundamental research on next-generation technology and radiotracer development in nuclear medicine (Figure 1.3).

The removal of funding with neither provision of bridge funding nor transfer of the research portfolio to another agency has created a sense of urgency about the need to assess the state of the science in nuclear medicine and to address two pre-existing problems that have been noted in other reports, namely (1) the critical shortage of trained chemists and clinical investigators in nuclear medicine and radiopharmaceutical science, and (2) the lack of a domestic source of radionuclides for research and development. To address uncertainties about whether and how future research in nuclear medicine should be funded, the DOE-OBER and the NIH jointly requested that the National Academies carry out this study and jointly sponsored this report.

The statement of task for this study (Sidebar 1.1) evolved out of discussions between the sponsoring agencies and the National Academies. Based on the discussions of the committee during the course of the study, the original fourth charge—to examine shortages of radiochemists—was expanded to include examination of shortages of highly trained nuclear medicine scientists.

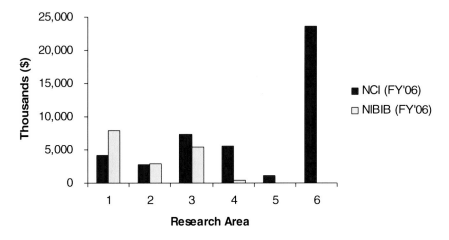

FIGURE 1.3 Breakdown of funding expended by NCI and NIBIB on nuclear medicine research by research area: 1 = Basic instrumentation development, 2 = Basic radiopharmaceutical development, 3 = Basic image reconstruction/analysis development, 4 = Development of new imaging procedures, 5 = Development of new therapy procedures, 6 = Clinical trials. SOURCE: Data provided by NCI and NIBIB.

1.1 STRATEGY TO ADDRESS THE STUDY CHARGE

The sponsors of the study requested that the National Academies produce a report for public dissemination within 13 months. This report fulfills that request.

The National Research Council of the National Academies appointed a committee of 14 experts to carry out this study. Biographical sketches of the committee members are provided in Appendix D. The committee met six times to gather information and develop this report. Details on the information-gathering sessions and speakers are provided in Appendix A. All of the information-gathering sessions were open to the public. Comments from interested organizations and individuals were encouraged and considered.

Within the specific scope outlined above, the committee reviewed information provided to it by members of the public, outside subject matter experts, scientific and medical societies, industry, and federal agencies. The committee made multiple requests for information from the DOE and the NIH. The committee was also able to access experts who could answer its technical questions. One meeting was devoted to perspectives from professional societies; another meeting focused on issues surrounding training of nuclear medicine personnel; and others were focused on gathering infor-

---

SIDEBAR 1.1 Statement of Task

The National Academies will perform a "state of the science" review of nuclear medicine and will provide findings and recommendations on the following issues

1.   Future needs for radiopharmaceutical development for the diagnosis and treatment of human disease (addressed in Chapters 3, 4, and 6).

2.   Future needs for computational and instrument development for more precise localization of radiotracers in normal and aberrant cell physiologies (addressed in Chapter 7).

3.   National impediments to the efficient entry of promising new radiopharmaceutical compounds into clinical feasibility studies and strategies to overcome them (addressed in Chapters 3, 4, 5, 6, and 8).

4.   Impacts of shortages of isotopes and highly trained radiopharmaceutical chemists and other nuclear medicine scientists on nuclear medicine basic and translational research, drug discovery, and patient care, and short- and long-term strategies to alleviate these shortages if they exist (addressed in Chapters 3 through 8).

In light of these future needs, the National Academies should examine the Medical Applications and Measurement Sciences Program and make recommendations to improve its research and isotope impacts on nuclear medicine. These recommendations should address both research thrusts and facility capabilities but should not address program management issues.

---

mation on the current state of the science of nuclear medicine and future directions of the field.

1.2 REPORT ROADMAP

The committee held extensive discussions about its interpretation of the statement of task (Sidebar 1.1) and the objective of the report. From these discussions, the committee determined that the primary focus of the report would be future opportunities in the field of nuclear medicine, within the context of the statement of task. The committee identified six specific issues originating from the statement of task, each of which is discussed in a separate chapter. The issues are:

- nuclear medicine imaging in diagnosis (Chapter 3);
- targeted radionuclide therapy (Chapter 4);
- radionuclide shortages (Chapter 5);
- radiopharmaceutical development (Chapter 6);
- computational and instrument development (Chapter 7); and

- training of nuclear medicine scientists and clinical investigators (Chapter 8).

Chapter 2 provides an overview of nuclear medicine as a discipline, which may be helpful to non-experts. It briefly summarizes important discoveries, challenges, and opportunities in the field. The appendixes provide supporting information, including a glossary and acronym list, descriptions of the committee's meetings, a list of commercially available radiopharmaceuticals, and biographical sketches of the committee members.

2

Nuclear Medicine

This chapter provides an overview of the field of nuclear medicine for readers who are not familiar with the discipline. It includes a description of the history and major discoveries in this field, the challenges of conducting nuclear medicine research, and the foreseeable new technologies and opportunities for personalizing health care that could result from aggressive development of the field.

Nuclear medicine is a highly multi-disciplinary specialty that develops and uses instrumentation and radiopharmaceuticals to study physiological processes and non-invasively diagnose, stage,[1] and treat diseases. A radiopharmaceutical is either a radionuclide alone, such as iodine-131 (Sidebar 2.1) or a radionuclide that is attached to a carrier molecule (a drug, protein, or peptide) or particle, which when introduced into the body by injection, swallowing, or inhalation accumulates in the organ or tissue of interest. In a nuclear medicine scan, a radiopharmaceutical is administered to the patient, and an imaging instrument that detects radiation is used to show biochemical changes in the body. Nuclear medicine imaging (Sidebar 2.2), in contrast to imaging techniques that mainly show anatomy (e.g., conventional ultrasound, computed tomography [CT], or magnetic resonance imaging [MRI]), can provide important quantitative functional information about normal tissues or disease conditions in living subjects. For treatment, highly targeted radiopharmaceuticals (Sidebar 2.3) may be used to deposit lethal radiation at tumor sites.

Nuclear medicine has been developed over the past 50 years through a

---

[1]Stage refers to a method of classifying patients by how far a disease has progressed.

SIDEBAR 2.1 Radionuclides Used in Nuclear Medicine

Radionuclides (also called radioisotopes) are chemical elements that are radioactive. The nucleus of an unstable radionuclide becomes stable by emitting energy, such as alpha or beta particles. The nucleus may also emit energy in the form of electromagnetic radiation known as gamma rays. Although radionuclides can be found in nature, all radionuclides used in nuclear medicine are produced in linear accelerators, cyclotrons, or nuclear reactors. Each radionuclide has unique properties that make it useful for certain diagnostic and therapeutic tools. The table summarizes commonly used radionuclides for imaging and therapy.

Commonly Used Radionuclides for Imaging and Therapy

Radionuclide	Half-Life	Type of Radiation Emitted	Imaging Technique Used
Imaging			
Carbon-11	20.33 min	positron	PET
Nitrogen-13	9.97 min	positron	PET
Oxygen-15	2.04 min	positron	PET
Fluorine-18	109.75 min	positron	PET
Technetium-99m	6.02 hours	gamma	SPECT
Indium-111	2.8 days	gamma	SPECT
Iodine-123	13 hours	gamma	SPECT
Therapy			
Iodine-131	8 days	beta	
Yttrium-90	2.7 days	beta	

unique partnership among the national laboratories, academia, and industry (Section 2.1). They have collaborated to develop:

- nuclear reactors and particle accelerators that produce radionuclides;
- chemical processes to synthesize radiopharmaceuticals that can be used for imaging and treatment; and
- instruments that can detect radiation emitted from the radionuclides that accumulate in the human body.

According to data from the Center for Medicare and Medicaid Services (CMS), nuclear medicine plays an essential role in medical specialties from cardiology to oncology to neurology and psychiatry and is a $1.7 billion industry. The Society of Nuclear Medicine estimates that 20 million nuclear

SIDEBAR 2.2 Nuclear Medicine Imaging

Positron emission tomography (PET) is a nuclear medicine imaging technique that exploits the unique decay physics of positron-emitting radionuclides (Sidebar 2.9) and produces a three-dimensional image of radionuclide distribution. For example, the radiopharmaceutical fluorine-18-fluorodeoxyglucose (FDG) is a form of sugar labeled with a radionuclide [fluorine-18] that is imaged using PET. This imaging technique, which is commonly known as FDG-PET, detects differences between cancer and normal cells in the consumption of glucose. Cancer cells, particularly those from aggressive tumors, proliferate more rapidly than normal cells and consume considerably larger amounts of glucose. Not only can tumor sites be pinpointed through the detection of increased FDG consumption, but differences in FDG consumption in tissues can be detected. However, FDG may be taken up by other lesions, such as infectious foci, and not just tumors, so the diagnostic specificity of FDG-PET is limited.

In the future, the network of cyclotron/radiopharmacies that are now focused exclusively on making FDG are well positioned to provide distribution of other fluorine-18-labeled radiopharmaceuticals to regional hospitals as these are developed and approved for clinical use. In addition, development and regional deployment of lower cost radionuclide-producing machines may make other radiopharmaceuticals based on radionuclides with shorter half-lives such as carbon-11 more widely available.

Single photon emission computed tomography (SPECT) is another common nuclear medicine imaging device. SPECT uses gamma cameras to obtain three-dimensional images. To acquire SPECT images, the gamma camera is rotated around the patient and multiple images from multiple angles are obtained. A computer can then reconstruct the images. Radiopharmaceuticals used for SPECT are labeled with gamma-emitting radionuclides such as technetium-99m, iodine-123, and thallium-201. SPECT is used extensively to study cardiac health (e.g., blood flow to the heart through myocardial perfusion imaging) and to image blood flow to the brain.

PET and SPECT each have distinct advantages and disadvantages that make them useful for detecting certain conditions. Each technique uses different properties of radioactive elements in creating an image. For example, one of the advantages of SPECT compared with PET is that more than one radiotracer can be used at a time. In addition, the longer half-life of radionuclides used with SPECT makes this imaging procedure more readily available to the medical community at large. However, PET images have higher sensitivity than SPECT images by a factor of 2 to 3 and use radiopharmaceuticals that provide more physiological information.

SIDEBAR 2.3 Targeted Radionuclide Therapy

Targeted radionuclide therapy is a form of treatment that delivers therapeutic doses of radiation to malignant tumors by administering a molecule that is labeled with a radionuclide. The radiotherapeutic agent is made of two components: the radionuclide and the carrier that is used to seek out the tumor cells. Molecular carriers that can be used include, but are not limited to, peptides that seek their corresponding receptors on cells, and monoclonal antibodies that seek out antigens that are similarly expressed on the cells, as shown in the figure.

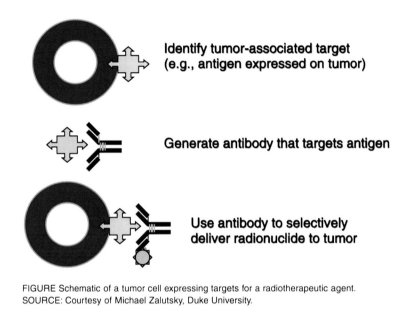

Identify tumor-associated target (e.g., antigen expressed on tumor)

Generate antibody that targets antigen

Use antibody to selectively deliver radionuclide to tumor

FIGURE Schematic of a tumor cell expressing targets for a radiotherapeutic agent.
SOURCE: Courtesy of Michael Zalutsky, Duke University.

The radionuclide that is attached to the carrier molecule can be chosen for specific characteristics, such as type of radiation decay (e.g., alpha-emitter, beta-emitter), radiation range, and half-life. It is this modular nature, where the two components can be varied like Lego® pieces to match characteristics specific to the tumor that makes targeted radionuclide therapy an attractive approach to cancer treatment (Zalutsky 2003). To date, two antibody radiopharmaceuticals have been approved by the FDA (yttrium-90-ibritumomab tiuxetan and iodine-131-tositumomab) for the treatment of lymphoma.

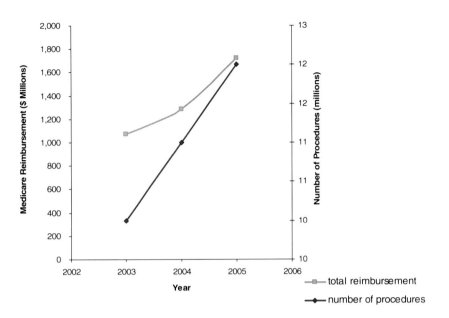

FIGURE 2.1 Number of nuclear medicine procedures that were approved for reimbursement by the Center for Medicare and Medicaid Services and total reimbursement for 2003–2005. SOURCE: Data provided by CMS.

medicine procedures are performed annually in the United States, of which 12 million are procedures approved for and reimbursed by CMS. Figure 2.1 illustrates the number of nuclear medicine procedures approved and the total payment reimbursed by the CMS in the United States in 2003, 2004, and 2005. Based on data from CMS, the use of positron emission tomography (PET) is growing faster than the use of any other imaging modality. From 2000 to 2005, the average annual growth rate in the volume of PET and PET/CT procedures was 80 percent compared with 9 percent for non-PET nuclear medicine procedures, 11 percent for CT, and 13 percent for MRI (ACR 2007). The use of nuclear medicine procedures will likely continue to rise in the future (Table 2.1).

More importantly, the use of nuclear medicine procedures has improved patient care in many ways. Nuclear imaging allows physicians to cost-effectively obtain medical information that would otherwise be unavailable or would require more invasive procedures, such as surgery or biopsy. For example, FDG-PET imaging has been estimated to save almost $400,000 per 100 patients when compared to surgery to assess for the presence of malignancy in indeterminate lung lesions as seen on CT (NLM 1998). This

TABLE 2.1 Procedures per Medicare Fee-for-Service Beneficiary, by Imaging Modality

	2000	2005	Average Annual Growth Rate (%)	Share of All Imaging (%) 2000	2005
All	3.83	4.99	5	100	100
CT	0.35	0.57	11	9	10
MRI	0.10	0.19	13	3	3
Nuclear Medicine					
Non-PET	0.21	0.33	9	5	6
PET and PET/CT	0.00	0.01	80	0.02	0.05
Ultrasound	0.84	1.14	6	22	22
Interventional	0.17	0.26	8	5	5
Mammography	0.21	0.33	9	6	6
X-ray, excluding mammography	1.94	2.14	2	51	49
Other	0.01	0.03	37	0.2	0.2

SOURCE: Data from American College of Radiology Research Department.

procedure, which has been in use for over 25 years, is also used to diagnose and stage esophageal cancer and non-small-cell lung cancer; to stage melanoma and colorectal cancers; and to monitor treatment response in lymphoma and locally advanced and metastatic breast cancer. FDG-PET has also had a considerable impact in detecting distant metastases and metastatic disease in lymph nodes that appear normal on CT scan (e.g., in lymphoma) (Kelloff et al. 2005).

2.1 SIGNIFICANT DISCOVERIES

The modern era of nuclear medicine is an outgrowth of the charge to the Atomic Energy Commission (AEC) "to exploit nuclear energy to promote human health" (Atoms for Peace Program). For more than 50 years, the AEC and later the Department of Energy (DOE) have supported high-risk research and development of nuclear medicine technology and have supplied radionuclides to the research community including physicists, chemists, engineers, computer scientists, biologists, and physicians. One of the earliest applications of nuclear medicine was the use of radioactive iodine to treat thyroid cancer. It also was used to measure thyroid function, diagnose thyroid disease, and treat hyperthyroidism, a condition where the thyroid gland produces excess amounts of thyroid hormones. The significant discoveries in nuclear medicine were made possible by advancements in the basic understanding of biological processes, chemistry, physics, and computer technology. Sidebar 2.4 lists the major breakthroughs resulting from past federal investment in nuclear medicine research.

2.2 FRONTIERS IN NUCLEAR MEDICINE

The output over the past 50 years, as documented in the preceding section, has been extensive. Although nuclear medicine already contributes to biomedical research and disease management, its promise is only beginning to be realized in areas such as neuroscience, drug development, preventive health care, and other aspects of medicine (Sidebar 2.5). Examples of advances that may be possible from continued multi-disciplinary research and development are discussed in the sections below. The first section (2.2.1) describes the various ways in which nuclear medicine can contribute to personalized health care. The second section (2.2.2) is devoted to the technologies currently under development that could enable advances in the field of nuclear medicine.

2.2.1 Opportunities in Personalizing Health Care

The knowledge gained and the tools developed during the course of the Human Genome Project[2] in addition to several decades of focused biomedical research are revolutionizing medicine. For example, thousands of genetic changes with known biological functions have been discovered and the number will grow as low-cost, next-generation genome analysis technologies are applied. This information will allow one to predict an individual's risk for disease, detect diseases earlier, predict disease outcome, and identify more effective treatments that will further personalize health care.

Disease Detection and Treatment Response

Omic[3] analyses are revealing differences in DNA, RNA, and protein expression between patients with cancer or heart disease and healthy subjects that can be detected in their blood, urine, feces, and sputum. Current tests are now approaching sensitivity levels that will allow detection of disease at subclinical levels, which is especially important for cancer management. Detection of subclinical disease demands the development of imaging procedures that can accurately pinpoint the location of the diseased tissue so

---

[2]The Human Genome Project was a 13-year international effort to determine the DNA sequence of human beings. It was initially conceived, proposed, and initiated by the DOE's Office of Biological and Environmental Research (DOE-OBER). The full sequence was completed in April 2003.

[3]Omic is an all-encompassing term used to describe comprehensive analyses of molecular or cellular characteristics. Genomics, for example, describes molecular assessment of the entire genome, and proteomics refers to measurement of the proteins found in cells and tissues.

SIDEBAR 2.4 Chronology of Significant Discoveries from Past Federal Funding

1930s

E.O. Lawrence at the UC Radiation Laboratory (later to become the Lawrence Berkeley National Laboratory) develops the cyclotron that will produce the first medically useful radionuclides, including iodine-131, thallium-201, technetium-99m, carbon-14, and gallium-67.

1940s

The first reactor-produced radionuclides for medical research are made at Oak Ridge National Laboratory (ORNL); these included phosphorous-32, iron-52, and chromium-51.

Carbon-11 was first produced and used in biological studies at the University of California at Berkeley by Martin Kamen and colleagues.

1950s

Benedict Cassen at the University of California at Los Angeles (UCLA) invents the first automated scanner to image the thyroid gland after administering radioiodine to patients.

Hal Anger invents the stationary gamma camera (now know as the Anger camera) at the UC Radiation Laboratory.

The molybdenum-99/technetium-99m generator is developed at Brookhaven National Laboratory (BNL) by Powell Richards. Today, technetium-99m is used in over 70 percent of nuclear medicine procedures worldwide (Nuclear Energy Agency 2000).

David Kuhl at the University of Pennsylvania constructs the prototype that will eventually lead to today's SPECT and CT scanners.

1960s

Scientists at ORNL discover the affinity of gallium-67 for soft-tissue tumors. This radionuclide has been used to image lymphomas, lung cancer, and brain tumors.

Hot atom chemistry[a] work by Alfred Wolf, Michael Welch, and other scientists lays the groundwork for what will become radiopharmaceutical chemistry.

William Eckelman and Powell Richards developed instant technetium kits.

1970s

The efficient production of thallium-201 is developed by scientists at BNL. This procedure is still used today to assess reduced blood flow or tissue damage to the heart.

PET scanners that will later be successfully commercialized are developed by Michael Phelps, Edward Hoffman, and Michel Ter-Pogossian at Washington University based on earlier work by Gordon Brownell at the Massachusetts Institute of Technology (MIT) and James Robertson at BNL.

Fluorine-18-FDG, a positron-emitting compound, is synthesized by chemists at BNL.

Scientists at the University of Pennsylvania and at the NIH use fluorine-18-FDG to image glucose metabolism in the human brain.

1980s
A new radiopharmaceutical, iodine-131 m-Iodine-benzyl-guanidine (I-131 MIBG), is developed by Donald Wieland for the diagnosis and treatment of rare childhood cancers.

Michael Welch of Washington University and John Katzenellenbogen of the University of Illinois develop the first PET radiotracer used to image tumors expressing the estrogen receptor.

Scientists at Harvard Medical School and MIT develop technetium-99m-methoxyisobutylnitrile, an agent to measure blood flow to the heart muscle (used in myocardial perfusion scans).

Chemists at national laboratories and federally supported academic laboratories developed methods to synthesize high-specific-activity C-11- and F-18-labeled compounds for imaging neurotransmitter and other physiological activities, laying the foundation for modern molecular imaging.

1990s
A high-resolution PET scanner designed to image small laboratory animals (i.e., microPET) is developed at UCLA by Simon Cherry.

Scientists at ORNL develop the rhenium-188 generator, which provides hospitals with a ready source of isotopes to treat bone pain in cancer patients.

Radionuclides (scandium-47, copper-67, samarium-153, rhenium-188, and gold-199) used in therapeutic nuclear medicine procedures are developed by scientists at multiple national laboratories.

Radiolabeled antibodies are developed for therapy (see Sidebar 2.3).

Advances are made in the application of alpha-particle emitters for therapy.

SOURCE: DOE 2001.

[a]Hot atom chemistry is the study of the chemical reactions that occur between high-energy atoms or molecules.

SIDEBAR 2.5 What is Personalized Medicine?

Personalized medicine refers to the tailoring of strategies to detect, treat, and prevent disease based on an individual's molecular characteristics (see examples below). Physicians already practice a form of personalized medicine by using diagnostic tests to choose treatment options; however, the wealth of knowledge that is emerging is helping physicians individualize treatment for each patient with greater precision (i.e., identify patients most likely to respond to a given treatment). Two examples, the second of which is specific to nuclear medicine, are provided to illustrate this concept.

Example 1: Trastuzumab (Herceptin®) as Treatment for Breast Cancer

Breast cancer is the most common form of cancer in women, after non-melanoma skin cancer and lung cancer, and approximately 180,000 new cases are diagnosed each year (CDC 2006). There are different types of breast cancer, and they are largely classified and treated on the basis of anatomy (i.e., which cells in the breast turn into cancer). More recently, with advances in the molecular characterization of the disease, oncologists now recognize that the subtypes of breast cancer are separate diseases that require different biologically based therapies.

One type of breast cancer overexpresses the human epidermal growth factor receptor 2 (HER2) receptor. An estimated 25 percent of breast cancer tumors are HER2-positive and these tumors tend to grow and spread more quickly compared with breast cancer tumors that are HER2-negative (Herceptin 2007). Trastuzumab, which is more commonly known under the trade name Herceptin®, is a monoclonal antibody that is designed to target breast tumors that express HER2. It is thought that trastuzumab stops the cancer cells from growing and dividing, and results from a large international clinical trial showed that the patients who received trastuzumab and chemotherapy were half as likely to have a recurrence of breast cancer as those who received chemotherapy alone (Piccart-Gebhard et al. 2005). This drug offers no benefit to patients whose breast cancer tumors do not overexpress HER2. By differentiating the tumors based on molecular differences and targeting these differences, more effective treatment can be delivered to the patient.

Example 2: Monitoring Response to Cancer Treatment with FDG-PET Imaging

FDG-PET is widely used in oncology to diagnose, stage, and restage[a] cancer. It is also used to detect residual cancer and to monitor the reduction in tumor

---

that it can be treated with a minimally invasive and, often, image-guided approach. The most exciting area in imaging today and going forward is molecular imaging through various imaging technologies from the laboratory setting to clinical research and practice. Molecular imaging has become a scientific discipline in its own right, as well as a growing practice in medicine. MRI and optical imaging, as well as nuclear medicine imaging, can be used for molecular targeting. The three approaches differ in sensitivity:

volume in response to therapy in cancer. Although its use for monitoring response is only reimbursed by Medicare for certain applications in the management of breast cancer, clinical trials in non-small-cell lung cancer, lymphoma, and esophageal cancer have shown that FDG-PET imaging can predict patient response to treatment. The figure below shows images taken in a lymphoma patient before and after treatment with the radioactively labeled anticancer agent, Zevalin. The tumor shows intense FDG uptake in the image taken before initiation of treatment. In contrast, the image taken after treatment shows a marked decrease in FDG uptake, indicating a favorable response to therapy. FDG-PET has the potential to improve patient care by allowing treatments with approved medicines to be selected to maximize individual patient response (Kelloff et al. 2005, Webber 2005).

---

[a]In oncology, restaging refers to reclassifying (i.e., staging) a patient's tumor after treatment has been initiated.

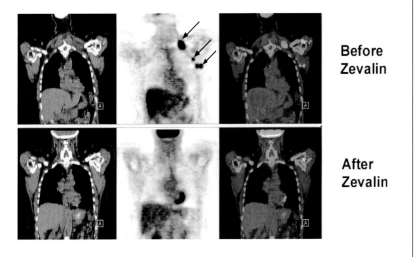

Before Zevalin

After Zevalin

FIGURE Monitoring response to treatment using FDG-PET in a lymphoma patient treated with Zevalin. SOURCE: courtesy of Peter Conti, University of Southern California.

MRI probes can be detected at micromolar concentrations, optical probes at picomolar concentrations, and nuclear probes at nanomolar concentrations. All of these probes can be chemically attached or encapsulated to target specific tissue receptor sites or may be attached to a moiety that preferentially accumulates in a region of interest. Nuclear photons, unlike optical ones, can escape from the body and thus can be used for more deeply seated targets (Weissleder 2006). It is therefore likely that nuclear medicine procedures can be developed to provide the precise information required to pinpoint the location of subclinical disease for minimally invasive treatment. This will require high-specific-activity radiotracers targeted to specific molecular markers as well as imaging devices with greater resolution and sensitivity.

"Omic" approaches are not only revealing previously unsuspected disease, but are also identifying subtypes of disease. The existence of disease subtypes may, in part, explain why similar clinical diagnoses often result in substantially different outcomes in different individuals. Nuclear medicine may contribute to the management of such diseases by providing information about individual responses to therapy. As illustrated in Sidebar 2.5, FDG-PET can be used to monitor responses of individual tumors to treatment by demonstrating whether there has been a change in FDG uptake. Such monitoring allows earlier determination of the effectiveness of approved treatments in individual patients and, if necessary, enables the patient to start an alternative treatment sooner. It also may facilitate evaluation of the effectiveness of experimental medicines, thereby speeding their entry into clinical practice while reducing cost. Other current as well as next-generation nuclear medicine procedures will similarly accelerate the delivery of personalized care to the patient.

Physiological Assessment

Nuclear medicine imaging will enable functional investigations of numerous aspects of normal and abnormal physiologies. These include, but are not limited to, neurotransmitter activity, chemical determinants of behavior, neurodegeneration, immune response, remodeling of heart tissue, and bone metabolism. Imaging of specific carbon-11-labeled agents to assess brain function is possible, but increasingly, fluorine-18-labeled compounds such as FDG, fluorine-18-dihydroxyphenylalanine, and fluorine-18-labeled fallypride[4] are being used to assess brain degeneration and cognitive function. Improvements in imaging instruments that have greater spatial and temporal resolution and radiotracers with high specific activities will allow more precise non-invasive assessment of these physiological functions. Ideally, next-generation procedures will use "natural" radionuclides such as carbon-11 that do not change the chemical properties of the tracer. In many cases, this will require imaging of low concentrations of proteins

---

[4] Fallypride is a chemical compound (i.e., benzamide) that binds specifically to the dopamine-2 and dopamine-3 receptors in the brain. Dopamine receptors have a role in processes such as motor and learning. Dysfunction in these receptors has been associated with a variety of neurological disorders, such as Parkinson's disease, schizophrenia, attention-deficit hyperactivity disorder, and drug dependence.

using radiotracers with short half-lives that have high specific activity. To achieve this, new technologies will need to be developed that can produce these short-half-life radionuclides cost-effectively at many sites distributed around the country (Section 2.2.2). Currently, they are available in research settings where a cyclotron and chemists are nearby.

Drug Development

The Pharmaceutical Research and Manufacturers of America (PHRMA 2006) reported for 2006 that 646 medicines were under development for cancer. This wealth of targets and therapeutic agents bodes well for individualized disease management. However, capitalizing on these developments requires years of work and considerable financial commitment. Using current approaches, the cost to bring a new drug to market is now estimated to be between $0.8 billion (DiMasi et al. 2003) and $1.7 billion (Mullin 2003) with a substantial risk of failure (Nunn 2006). In part, this is because only one in five drugs that enter clinical trials actually proceeds to an approval stage (Wierenga and Eaton 2007), and many drugs fail in the late stages of clinical testing (i.e., phase II or III), after a considerable amount of money has been spent. Moreover, the time line for bringing a new drug to clinical use takes, on average, 12 years (Wierenga and Eaton 2007).

The time and expense required to bring a drug to market may be reduced by using nuclear medicine imaging technologies to identify which drugs should advance from animal to human studies, reveal mechanisms of drug action, evaluate drug distribution to target tissue; establish the drug occupancy of receptor sites; assess the actions of new agents on specific molecular targets or pathways; and determine appropriate dose range and regimen (Eckelman 2003). It has been estimated that the use of PET during Phase I studies (Sidebar 2.6) could save upward of $235 million in research and drug development costs (Phelps 2006) for each successful drug. It is anticipated that the drug development process will be facilitated by the availability of molecularly targeted radiopharmaceuticals, high-resolution PET/CT and PET/MRI imaging machines, and image quantification software. With this in mind, the Oncology Biomarker Qualification Initiative, through cooperation among big Pharma, the Food and Drug Administration (FDA), the National Cancer Institute (NCI), and CMS, has begun to foster qualification of molecular imaging endpoints (FDA 2006b). The overall approach will bring together the strengths of these three agencies and the pharmaceutical industry to determine the optimum use of biomarkers to evaluate treatment response. Clearly, radiotracers are likely to be excellent biomarkers. For example, the NCI has begun the development of task forces to plan joint trials based on PET/CT with the goal of qualifying FDG as a biomarker in non-small-cell lung cancer and in lymphoma.

SIDEBAR 2.6 Introduction to Clinical Trials

A clinical trial is a research study conducted in human volunteers that is designed to answer specific questions. There are different types of clinical trials, such as treatment, prevention, diagnostic, and screening trials, each of which answers a different question. Treatment trials are the most common, and clinical trials are conducted in phases, where each phase has a different purpose.

Phase I trials: An experimental drug or treatment is given to a small group of patient volunteers (usually between 20 and 80) to evaluate its safety, determine a safe dosage range, and identify side effects.

Phase II trials: The experimental drug is given to a larger group of patient volunteers (typically 100 to 300) to determine whether it is effective and to further evaluate its safety.

Phase III trials: The effectiveness of the experimental drug is confirmed when compared to commonly used treatments in large groups of patient volunteers. Sample size largely depends on the anticipated effect size from the treatments being compared and the size needed to detect a difference. Typically, phase III trials have several hundred to several thousand patient volunteers. Side effects and safety in patients continue to be monitored.

Phase IV trials (also known as post-marketing studies): These studies are conducted to collect additional information on the drug's risks and benefits that may not have emerged during the previous studies.

SOURCE: NIH 2006.

Furthermore, the value of molecular imaging in drug discovery and development has been recognized by big Pharma with nearly 65 percent of drugs losing their patent protection by 2010, which represents a $70 billion loss in revenue per year. Merck, Glaxo, Pfizer, Bristol-Myers-Squibb, Genentech, and Johnson and Johnson are among the companies with active in-house or collaborative programs for conducting radiotracer imaging as a guide to drug discovery and development. The types of studies being conducted relate to both pharmacokinetics, through labeling of drugs of interest, and pharmacodynamics, using molecular imaging for key processes (e.g., glycolysis, proliferation, and hypoxia) fundamental to oncology and other medical specialties, as ways to observe the effects of drugs in vivo. In some of the larger programs, such as those of Merck and Glaxo, the staff is measured in the dozens, and includes nuclear medicine physicians, medicinal chemists, kineticists, radiochemists, pharmacologists, and imaging technicians.

Imaging development is often in the context of the broad capabilities

of molecular imaging and may include magnetic resonance and spectroscopy, bioluminescence and fluorescence imaging, but nuclear imaging plays
a prominent role. In part, this is because of major advances in enabling
technology, such as microPET and microSPECT (single positron emission
computed tomography), with resolution in the 1-mm range that is suitable
for experiments and small laboratory animals. New molecules under development are often chemically designed for easy radiolabeling to facilitate
the production of representative radiotracers for pharmacological bioavailability and pharmacodynamic studies. Radiotracers developed in this way
are often initially studied in animals, with straightforward pharmacology
studies seamlessly translated to human volunteers using PET/CT high-resolution imaging.

Also, in the past few years, medical imaging instrument companies
have teamed up with radiopharmaceutical development groups, within both
industry and academia, to foster radiopharmaceutical development for the
rapidly growing market in PET/CT and SPECT/CT. General Electric acquired Amersham, a large radiopharmaceutical company. Siemens acquired
CTI, including PET-NET, which is a network of radiopharmacies involved
in distributing positron emitters and single photon emitters to nuclear
medicine practitioners within hospitals. Phillips has developed numerous
collaborations with academic institutions in both Europe and the United
States in molecular imaging.

In companies that develop neuroleptic drugs, there has been a heavy
emphasis on pharmacokinetic and pharmacodynamic studies directed at
evaluating saturation of key receptors in vivo. These studies are being done
because of the recognition that doses that are greater than those required
to saturate the target neuroreceptor simply result in more neurotoxicity
without beneficial effects. For example, the dopamine D2 receptor binding
agent carbon-11-racalopride may be used as a radiotracer for the dopamine
D2 receptor, and a novel new drug intended for use in schizophrenia, with
high affinity for the D2 receptor, may be used in conjunction with the radiotracer to find optimal dosage regimens in humans that will just saturate
the dopamine D2 receptor, as shown by the displacement of carbon-11-
racalopride. In this way, the optimal biologic dosage may be used without
running the risk of binding to collateral receptor targets in the brain and
producing undesirable toxicity.

Targeted Radiotherapeutics

Therapeutic nuclear medicine procedures are now used to treat thyroid
cancer and other thyroid disorders, relieve pain from bone metastases, or

---

**SIDEBAR 2.7 Scientific Fields Expanding
Nuclear Medicine Capabilities**

Nanotechnology is a broad scientific field that creates and uses materials and devices that are so small they are measured in nanometers. One nanometer is one-billionth of a meter. Although application of this technology is still limited, it is expected to change the computer industry and medical practice (NNI 2007).

Materials science is an inter-disciplinary field comprising applied physics, chemistry, and engineering that studies the physical properties of matter and its applications.

Microfluidics is a multi-disciplinary field that studies how fluids behave at microliter and nanoliter volumes and stimulates the design of systems in which small volumes of fluids are used to provide automated sample processing, synthesis, separation, and measurements in devices commonly described by the term "lab-on-a-chip" (see Chapter 6). For example, microfluidics is used in DNA analysis.

---

treat blood disorders such as lymphoma and polycythemia vera.[5] Research programs and clinical trials are currently underway to address the utility of molecularly targeted radionuclide therapies in treating rheumatoid arthritis, degenerative joint diseases, heart disease, non-small-cell lung cancer, colon cancer, prostate cancer, pancreatic cancer, ovarian cancer, meningitis, and AIDS. However, this is only the beginning. Information from large-scale omic analyses stimulated by the Cancer Genome Atlas Project[6] and from focused molecular studies being conducted throughout the scientific community may reveal many new tumor-specific molecules through which therapeutic doses of radiation can potentially be delivered. New carrier molecules exploiting nanotechnologies and other advances in materials science (Sidebar 2.7) may further increase the efficacy of targeted radiotherapeutics. It is envisioned that treatments that are specific to a patient will be developed. For example, depending on the characteristics of a tumor, a variety of radionuclides, carrier molecules, and molecular targets (see Sidebar 2.3) could be used to maximize treatment efficacy and minimize normal tissue toxicity. Targeted radionuclide therapy is further discussed in Chapter 7.

---

[5]Polycythemia vera is a blood disorder where there is an overproduction of red blood cells, white blood cells, and platelets. Patients with this disorder are prone to developing clots that can result in strokes or heart attacks.

[6]The Cancer Genome Atlas Project is an interdisciplinary program established and administered by the NCI (NCI 2007a) and the National Human Genome Research Institute. Its goal is to comprehensively measure changes in DNA sequence, genome copy number, allelotype, gene expression, and methylation in normal and cancer cells in order to identify abnormalities that influence cancer genesis and progression.

2.2.2 Enabling Technologies

The future of nuclear medicine depends on the development of enabling technologies in several areas. These include technologies that will cost-effectively increase access to radionuclides, miniaturize the chemical process that will make it possible to produce multiple different radiopharmaceuticals to meet pre-clinical and clinical demands, and increase the speed and resolution of SPECT, PET, and combined-modality imaging.

Compact Devices to Generate Radionuclides with Short Half-Lives

One of the principal obstacles to realizing the full potential of nuclear medicine in advancing medical science and patient care is the limited accessibility of radionuclides with short half-lives (i.e., less than 30 minutes). Although these radionuclides have numerous advantages (Sidebar 2.8),

---

SIDEBAR 2.8 Advantages of Radionuclides with Short Half-Lives

Carbon, nitrogen, oxygen, and fluorine are common elements found in biologically active molecules and pharmaceuticals. The use of the radionuclides carbon-11, nitrogen-13, and oxygen-15 as replacements for non-radioactive carbon, nitrogen, and oxygen provides radioactive compounds with the exact same chemical and biological properties as the non-radioactive compounds. As carbon is abundant in biologically active molecules, the replacement of carbon-12 by carbon-11 provides a convenient way to produce many tracers and drugs where the properties of the parent carbon-12 molecule are well-established. There are many examples of carbon-11 compounds that have been developed. They have been used to study carbohydrate and lipid metabolism, receptors and enzymes in the brain, and drug pharmacokinetics.[a]

Carbon-11 (half-life = 20 min), nitrogen-13 (half-life =10 min) and oxygen-15 (half-life = 2 min) are all positron emitters with short half-lives. Short-lived radionuclides have several advantages. The absorbed radiation dose to the patient being studied is generally less than with a longer-lived tracer, allowing more tracer to be injected. In turn, the higher amount of tracer increases the signal that the imaging instrument can detect. Furthermore, several studies may be performed on the same patient on the same day since the tracer radioactivity decays quickly. Despite their versatility, their short half-lives limit their use to institutions that are near facilities that can rapidly synthesize and purify radiotracer compounds so that imaging studies can be completed before the radioactivity decays.

---

[a]Pharmacokinetics is a branch of pharmacology that studies what the body does with a drug (e.g., how it is absorbed, distributed, metabolized, and excreted).

their use dictates that imaging be performed near the facility in which the radionuclide is produced. The current supply is from a few cyclotrons that are primarily used to produce fluorine-18. The initial investment for such a cyclotron is $2 million, with an additional $0.5 million needed for renovation and installation. At a minimum, another $0.8 million is needed to cover annual operating costs,[7] assuming no major repairs are needed (personal communication, Thomas Budinger, Lawrence Berkeley National Laboratory, July 2, 2007). Consideration could be given to developing a low-cost, low-maintenance accelerator that would be in the category of a tabletop instrument. Some design specifications for a compact generator that might be developed include a miniature linear proton accelerator using modern engineering and new target designs, acceleration of helium-3 atoms into a primary target doped with deuterium to produce 15 MeV protons, photonuclear-based isotope production, and laser-stimulated proton production. Shielding and minimization of external radiation would have to be incorporated into its design.

Nanotechnology and Microfluidics

Remarkable advances are now being made in materials science and microfluidics that provide unique opportunities in nuclear medicine. Miniaturization of radiochemical production systems has the potential to improve reaction yields, increase cost-effectiveness, and expand access to the products to more users. These smaller devices in combination with compact radionuclide generators may facilitate the production of multiple radiopharmaceuticals to meet the pre-clinical and clinical demands of researchers and physicians. The miniaturization of the chemistry will make it possible to reduce radiation shielding requirements and further simplify the required infrastructure for preparing the radiopharmaceuticals. New chemical reagents, such as polymer-supported precursors, may also be used to produce cleaner, higher specific-activity tracers. Increased specific activity and decreased impurities will assist with FDA approval of tracers.

Scintillator[8] Crystals and Semiconductors

Both PET and SPECT depend on multi-element radiation detectors to produce anatomic images of radionuclide distribution (Sidebar 2.9). The images achieved in current instruments are degraded by radiation scattering

---

[7]Annual operating costs include salaries for a full-time cyclotron technician, a full-time radiopharmacist, a half-time radiochemist, supplies, service contracts, and overhead.

[8]A scintillator is a substance that absorbs energy of charged particle radiation or gamma radiation and then releases this energy through fluorescence.

within the body.[9] Detection of this scatter can be decreased substantially by improving the energy resolution of multi-element radiation detectors used in imaging. This can be accomplished by developing detectors that have increasing radiation detection efficiency (photoelectric absorption), short timing resolution, good energy resolution, high luminosity, and low dead time. Next-generation fast, high-efficiency scintillators are now being developed to support homeland security applications that are intended to have this optimum combination of detector properties. These new detector materials will substantially improve nuclear medicine imaging when incorporated into next-generation PET and SPECT devices.

Combined-Modality Imaging (PET/CT, PET/MRI, and SPECT/CT)

CT, MRI, and PET all provide complementary "views" of normal and diseased tissues, with PET offering quantitative functional information and MRI and CT scans providing high-resolution anatomical information. The power of combined-modality imaging will increase dramatically as molecularly targeted radiotracers with high specific activity are developed and as the sensitivity and resolution of PET increase to allow for high-resolution, temporal imaging. The simple methods developed in the 1970s for image reconstruction in microscopy are no longer sufficient for reconstructing images taken with PET and SPECT. The images are reconstructed using iterative procedures that take into account the relationship between the image space and the detector or projection space. The connection between the two is known as the system matrix. In modern imaging technologies, the system matrix becomes quite large, and currently, the computational speed and memory of commercial computers are inadequate. Full realization of the potential of combined-modality imaging will emerge as computational techniques are developed to manage noise (i.e., increase the signal-to-background ratio) and improve segmentation,[10] feature recognition, and multimodality image registration.[11]

---

[9]Scattering is a physical process in which particles are deflected from their paths through interactions with other particles.

[10]Image segmentation is a procedure that allows for unwanted structures in the image to be removed.

[11]Data taken from a given patient at different points in time or from different angles need to be transformed so comparisons can be made. Image registration is the process by which the different measurements are integrated.

SIDEBAR 2.9 Introduction to the Physics of PET

A radiotracer that is labeled with a positron-emitting radionuclide, such as fluorine-18, is injected into the patient undergoing a PET scan. The radionuclides then decay, emitting positrons. The resulting positrons subsequently annihilate on contact with electrons within the body (Figure 1). Each annihilation event produces two photons traveling in opposite directions that are detected by the detectors surrounding the patient. If this detection occurs within a certain time, it is considered to have come from the same annihilation event and is "coincident" (Figure 2).

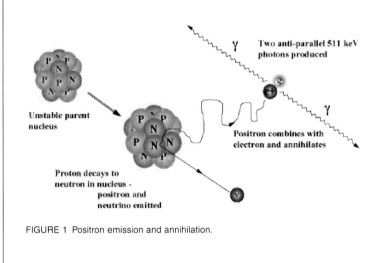

FIGURE 1 Positron emission and annihilation.

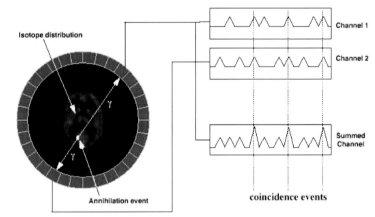

FIGURE 2 Schematic of coincidence event detection.

In PET, there are four types of coincidence events: true, scattered, random, and multiple. Figure 3 illustrates the first three. A coincidence event is assigned to a line of response (LOR). In this way, positional information is gained from the radiation that is detected.

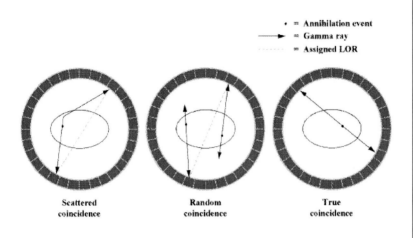

FIGURE 3 Types of coincidences.

Time-of-flight means that for each annihilation event the precise time that each of the coincident photons is detected is noted and the difference in arrival time is calculated. Since the closer photon will arrive at the detector first, calculating the difference in arrival time helps determine the location of the annihilation event between the two detectors. Theoretically, perfect time-of-flight information would eliminate the need to reconstruct images. However, even the addition of imperfect time-of-flight information reduces noise and improves the image by approximating the location of the annihilation event. This improvement in image quality is particularly useful in large patients (Badawi 1999, Karp 2006).

2.3 COMPLEXITIES OF NUCLEAR MEDICINE PRACTICE AND RESEARCH

The field of nuclear medicine is multi-disciplinary, and successful development and delivery of these potentially life-saving procedures to patients involves specialists from clinical fields such as radiology, nuclear medicine, cardiology, oncology, psychiatry, infectious disease, surgery, and endocrinology, collaborating with imaging specialists, engineers, computer scientists, physicists, chemists, and molecular biologists.

As described above, the developments in nuclear medicine over the past 50 years have been extensive and the future is bright. However, for the field to flourish, there are scientific, regulatory, and financial obstacles that need to be addressed. Section 2.3.1 describes the basic science research challenges; Section 2.3.2 summarizes clinical research challenges; Section 2.3.3 summarizes the regulatory hurdles and explores the costs and economics of the field; and Section 2.3.4 discusses radiation exposure from nuclear medicine procedures and its relative safety.

2.3.1 Basic Science Research Challenges

Most of the significant developments in nuclear medicine during the past 50 years have leveraged the substantial engineering and physical sciences infrastructure that was developed to support research in nuclear physics, neutron science, and nuclear power technologies, which included, but were not limited to nuclear power production and nuclear propulsion. For example, the nuclear reactors used to produce radionuclides were developed primarily in support of research directed toward nuclear power generation. Similarly, cyclotrons used to produce medical radionuclides were developed using technologies that were originally invented to support particle physics research. This is also true for the scintillator detectors and electronics used in PET imaging. In addition, these technological advancements were the result of work spanning several decades. Long-term investments that could sustain multi-disciplinary teams were necessary to allow for the time needed to develop new concepts using insights from the fields of physics, chemistry, and materials science; to identify areas of biology or medicine where these concepts might be applied; and to develop practical devices or reagents that could be tested in the biological or clinical setting.

Today, the substantial nuclear physics research infrastructure that spawned many developments in nuclear medicine has diminished considerably. It has been offset to some extent by research infrastructure being developed to support efforts in biofuels[12] research, homeland security, and

---

[12]Biofuel is a renewable energy source that is composed of biological material. An example of a biofuel is ethanol.

nanotechnology. However, the financial support needed to sustain research in nuclear physics and these new fields to advance nuclear medicine has been reduced, and the funding that remains is generally awarded to small teams of scientists for short durations. As a consequence, research teams focus predominantly on short-term proof-of-principle experiments and not on sustained development of practical instruments or radiotracer chemistry methods. This change in research focus has substantially impeded the development of next-generation technologies in nuclear medicine that could potentially allow more personalized health care.

2.3.2 Clinical Research Challenges

Beyond the need for greater inter-disciplinary cooperation, the field of nuclear medicine faces other challenges that are unique to it. Investigators face regulatory hurdles in the investigational new drug (IND) application process[13] (explored further in Section 2.3.3), limited isotope availability (Chapter 5), and a shortage of expertise in radiopharmaceutical chemistry, radiopharmacy (Chapter 8), and image acquisition and interpretation. All of these are barriers to bringing novel imaging agents, radio-therapeutics, and devices to the clinical environment.

Assuming that animal studies of a new diagnostic or therapeutic radio-pharmaceutical produce encouraging results and that studies in humans can begin, the field is currently limited by a lack of standardization and coordination in clinical trials. In the field of targeted radionuclide therapy, for example, there are currently too many individual clinical trials enrolling too few patients and treating them in widely varying ways. Similarly, clinical trials for diagnostic imaging suffer from different clinical centers using different imaging platforms. This has led to a lack of uniformity in how data are acquired, handled, stored, and interpreted. Building on the experience of cooperative groups, such as the American College of Radiology Imaging Network (ACRIN 2007) and the U.S. FDA, it is important that investigational approaches be standardized so that data can be compared across clinical trials and translated into clinical practice.

2.3.3 Regulatory Hurdles and Costs

Regulatory requirements pose additional hurdles to translational research and clinical investigations. In the United States, all pharmacologic

---

[13]During drug development, promising candidates are selected using in vitro models. Candidates that are not rejected are then tested in in vivo animal models. After toxicological data have been collected and basic safety tests have been performed in animals, an IND must be submitted to the FDA before testing in human subjects can begin in a phase I study (see Sidebar 2.6).

agents, including diagnostic radiopharmaceuticals and radiotherapeutics, undergo regulatory oversight by the FDA. However, radiopharmaceuticals face additional scrutiny and have unique regulatory and approval pathways. At times, the requirements, such as extensive toxicology testing, have been unpredictable, posing considerable financial burdens that are frequently beyond the means of investigators in academia. There are concerns that these regulatory hurdles have impeded translational research to the extent that some major clinical investigations have migrated from the United States to other countries with less demanding requirements.

For example, obtaining an IND to permit clinical evaluation of a promising targeted radiotherapeutic agent requires toxicology data and information on pharmacokinetics and dosimetry of the radiopharmaceutical (FDA 2005). Furthermore, radiochemistry methods frequently need significant modification and optimization in order to be able to reliably supply the labeled drug at the activity levels needed for patient treatment. Because this is generally not hypothesis-driven research, it is difficult to obtain grant support for it. Unlike the Development of Clinical Imaging Drugs and Enhancers program (NCI 2007b), which can help offset the costs of some of these studies for imaging agents, there is no analogous mechanism available for targeted radiotherapeutics.

In an effort to reduce some of the regulatory hurdles, the FDA issued guidance to the research community on the exploratory Investigational New Drug (eIND)[14] process (FDA 2006a). The stated goal of eIND studies is to reduce the time and resources expended on candidate products that are unlikely to succeed. Although the introduction of eINDs has aided in bringing new radiotracers, it is too early to determine whether the stated goal will be achieved.

An academic research base is necessary to allow industry to rise to the challenge of delivering novel technology for future clinical use. For clinical trials to be successful, industry must be engaged and see a clear pathway for economic success. Industry will not develop the technology necessary to deploy the next generation of genome-based medicines unless the scientific and economic rationale has been identified by academia.

---

[14]In its March 2004 Critical Path Report, the FDA stated that new tools were needed to distinguish earlier in the drug development process which candidates hold promise and which ones do not. Because only 8 percent of new medical compounds entering phase I testing reach the market, the FDA established eIND studies as a way of trying to reduce the time and cost of drug development. In an eIND study, the goal is to verify results observed in experimental models in humans and determine pharmacological properties rather than determine dose-limiting toxicities. Because eIND studies present fewer potential risks than do traditional phase I studies, they may reduce the number of human subjects and resources needed to identify promising drugs.

2.3.4 Radiation Exposure and Safety

There has been greater awareness recently that medical imaging procedures, especially interventional, CT, and nuclear medicine tests, contribute significantly to the annual collective radiation dose (AMA 2006, NCRP 2007, Amis et al. 2007). In the past 25 years, medical radiation exposure has risen from about 15 percent to greater than 50 percent of the total annual exposures to the U.S. population. For the currently estimated medical collective dose of 930,000 person-Sieverts (Sv), 23 percent derives from nuclear medical procedures, of which 85 percent are cardiac examinations. The individual (effective) dose for a rest and exercise cardiac study using a technetium-99m-labeled agent is ~10mSv and is estimated to produce an approximate radiation-induced cancer risk of 0.05 percent in a naturally healthy individual against a background cancer rate of approximately 40 percent (NRC 2006). Given the age and infirmity of the group undergoing cardiac studies, this risk estimate is undoubtedly overestimated. Nonetheless, indications for such procedures need to be deemed to have a medical benefit and continued efforts must be made to reduce the absorbed radiation dose without sacrificing diagnostic accuracy. In 2006, the American Medical Association House of Delegates adopted a directive, in collaboration with specialty societies and interested stakeholders, "(a) to examine the feasibility of monitoring and quantifying the cumulative radiation exposure sustained by individual patients in medical settings; and (b) to discuss methods to educate physicians and the public on the appropriate use and risks of low linear energy transfer radiation in order to reduce unnecessary exposure in the medical setting."

The increasing use of FDG-PET scanning, which provides approximately the same absorbed dose to patients as cardiac studies, deserves similar considerations as well as raises some additional concerns given the higher energy of annihilation (positron-producing) photons. Shielding and other measures need to be employed in order to protect radiation personnel, families, and bystanders (Madsen et al. 2006) and need to be incorporated into contemporary clinical and preparatory facilities.

Radiopharmaceuticals are administered in small mass amounts, generally nanomoles, so as to follow the tracer principle. Consequently, imaging agents have little or no pharmacologic effect. Furthermore, the tracer activities employed in nuclear medicine diagnostic procedures result in radiation doses well below the threshold for any acute (deterministic) radiation toxicity. The incidence of misadministration has been extremely low in the past (NCRP 1991). With the promulgation of even stricter rules of the Joint Commission on Accreditation of Healthcare Organizations on monitoring of all prescribed substances to patients, new measures aimed to lessen patient, staff, and family radiation exposures to offset the trend set by the increasing number of diagnostic procedures is to be expected.

2.4 CONCLUSION

We have arrived at a crossroads in nuclear medicine. Further development of the field will likely contribute substantially to the development of personalized medicine by (1) providing more efficient and lower cost strategies to bring new drugs to market; (2) developing new and more effective treatments for cancer and cardiovascular disease; (3) improving understanding of abnormal physiological conditions; and (4) developing new, effective anticancer drugs. Moreover, new developments in accelerator engineering, computer science, materials science, chemistry, and nanotechnology suggest that a new generation of nuclear medicine instruments and radiopharmaceuticals can now be made that will be less expensive, more widely available, and more precise. Although there are challenges ahead, by investing in the infrastructure of radionuclide production; committing to train and nurture the next generation of nuclear medicine researchers, technicians, and clinicians; and developing a program that will sustain nuclear medicine research, we will all reap the benefits of better health care.

3

Nuclear Medicine Imaging in Diagnosis and Treatment

In this chapter, we describe the role of nuclear medicine imaging in patient care and review how these imaging approaches contribute to the diagnosis of disease, to the assessment of the disease-related risk to patients, and to individualizing treatment strategies for improving patient outcomes and survival. The chapter is organized into the following sections:

- Background (3.1),
- Current State of Nuclear Medicine Imaging and Emerging Priorities (3.2), and
- Impediments to Progress and Current and Future Needs (3.3).

3.1 BACKGROUND

Nuclear medicine imaging non-invasively provides functional information at the molecular and cellular level that contributes to the determination of health status by measuring the uptake and turnover of target-specific radiotracers in tissue. These functional processes include tissue blood flow and metabolism, protein—protein interactions, expression of cell receptors in normal and abnormal cells, cell—cell interactions, neurotransmitter activity, cell trafficking and homing, tissue invasion, and programmed cell death. By providing information on these processes, nuclear medicine imaging offers a broad array of tools for probing normal and disease-related states of tissue function and response to treatment.

The addition of anatomic imaging provided by computed tomography (CT) to functional imaging of positron emission tomography (PET) and single photon emission computed tomography (SPECT) has further expanded the utility and accuracy of nuclear medicine imaging. By using combined-modality PET/CT and SPECT/CT devices, functional processes can be localized within the body to an anatomically identified or, in some instances, as yet unidentifiable structural alteration. These devices have enhanced the accuracy with which disease can be detected, aided in the determination of the extent and severity of disease, enhanced the accuracy for identifying disease-related risk, and improved the ability to monitor patient response to therapy.

3.2 CURRENT STATE OF NUCLEAR MEDICINE IMAGING AND EMERGING PRIORITIES

This section describes the use of nuclear medicine imaging for three types of diseases to illustrate its impact on patient diagnosis and management and to identify emerging priorities. The three types of disease are cancer (Section 3.2.1), cardiovascular disease (Section 3.2.2), and neurological disorders (e.g., Alzheimer's disease) (Section 3.2.3). In addition, the use of nuclear medicine imaging in drug development is discussed in Section 3.2.4.

3.2.1 Cancer

Cancer develops when cells begin to divide out of control. One hallmark of cancer cells is that they consume larger amounts of glucose than normal cells, because of a shift in energy production. This shift is known as "the Warburg effect" (Sidebar 3.1). Fluorine-18-fluorodeoxyglucose (FDG)-

---

SIDEBAR 3.1 The Warburg Effect

Cells generate energy in two main ways: oxidative phosphorylation in mitochondria and glycolysis in the cytoplasm. In oxidative phosphorylation, 38 adenosine triphosphate (ATP) molecules[a] are generated per glucose molecule. In contrast, two ATP molecules are produced per glucose molecule through glycolysis (a less efficient way of generating energy that requires a greater amount of glucose to produce the same number of ATP molecules). Although cells use both pathways, they primarily switch to glycolysis at times of oxygen deprivation. Nobel Prize-winning German biochemist Otto Warburg observed that cancer cells preferentially generate energy through glycolysis, even in the presence of oxygen. This phenomenon is known as the Warburg effect (Garber 2004).

---

[a]ATP is the main energy source for cellular function.

PET (Sidebar 2.2) has exploited this feature of cancer cells to detect differences between cancer and normal cells in the consumption of glucose. The accumulation of FDG in cancer cells represents an in vivo correlate of the abnormal mitochondrial function found in many types of cancer cells. Differences in rate of glucose utilization distinguish malignant from benign tumors and identify the presence and spread of tumor metastases as measures of disease severity. This information is important for tumor staging and for designing therapeutic strategies.

There is increasing evidence that imaging with FDG-PET may have an even greater impact on patient management as a way of monitoring tumor response to therapy (Juweid and Cheson 2006, Weber and Wieder 2006). Changes in glucose consumption can be detected using FDG-PET, where a reduction in tumor uptake of FDG predicts the likely effectiveness of chemotherapy. As Figure 3.1 illustrates, a favorable response can be

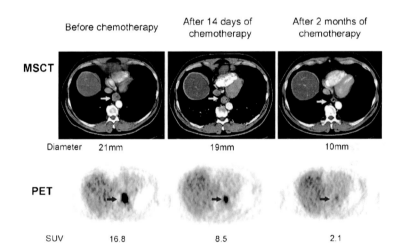

FIGURE 3.1 Monitoring the effects of chemotherapy on tumor volume and glucose uptake with serial multislice computed tomography (MSCT) and PET imaging in a patient with cancer of the esophagus. Imaging was performed before the start of treatment (left), 2 weeks after the start of chemotherapy (middle), and again after 2 months (right). The large tumor seen on the MSCT image (yellow arrow) is associated with intense FDG uptake on the pre-treatment PET image (red arrow). At 2 weeks, the tumor volume decreased only mildly (decrease in diameter from 21 mm to 19 mm), while the FDG uptake declined by about 50 percent (reflected by the decrease in the standardized uptake value of FDG from 16.8 to 8.5). At 3 months, the tumor volume has strikingly decreased and the FDG uptake is only faintly visible. SOURCE: Reprinted by permission of the Society of Nuclear Medicine from Wieder et al. 2005.

detected by PET, but not with CT, as early as 2 weeks from initiation of chemotherapy in a patient with esophageal cancer (Wieder et al. 2005). At 2 weeks, the tumor volume as measured with CT had decreased minimally (diameter from 21 mm to 19 mm), while the FDG uptake had declined by about 50 percent. At 3 months, the tumor volume has strikingly decreased and the FDG uptake is only faintly visible. By contrast, in patients where there is a persistent high uptake of FDG, the absence of a therapeutic response is noted. Therefore, early assessment of tumor response to therapy with FDG-PET has the potential to considerably reduce the side effects and costs of ineffective therapies.

As noted above, tumor imaging with FDG-PET has been clinically useful in oncology because it captures the increased rate of glucose utilization. Yet, its utility has some limitations due to organ-specific utilization of glucose. For example, its use in diagnosing prostate and liver cancers has been limited due to the low metabolic activities of these cancers. The brain, in contrast, uses glucose for normal function. This characteristic has made it difficult to delineate tumors from normal brain tissue by FDG-PET. Similarly, increased glucose utilization is also observed when the body responds to damage (i.e., inflammation). Therefore, certain inflammatory processes cannot be differentiated from tumor tissue by FDG-PET.

However, depending on the radiotracer used, PET provides diagnostic information based on other types of metabolic activity, such as amino acid[1] metabolism, cell proliferation, and tissue hypoxia.[2] For example, amino acids and amino acid analogs[3] have been labeled with fluorine-18 or carbon-11 and have been reported to be superior to FDG for imaging of brain tumors (Pirotte et al. 2004, Nariai et al. 2005, W. Chen et al. 2006). Another class of PET tracers that has shown promise is radiolabeled thymidine analogs (Shields 2006). The use of these tracers is based on the hypothesis that they mimic the biological behavior of thymidine, and thereby provide a measurement of DNA synthesis and cell proliferation in vivo. By extension, these tracers provide an accurate measure of tumor growth (Shields et al. 1998). Analogues of thymidine such as fluorine-18-fluoro-L-thymidine and fluorine-18-1-(2'-deoxy-2'-fluoro-β-darabinofuranosyl) thymine, also are being investigated as potential agents for monitoring early response to therapy.

Another promising application of PET is the use of probes, such as fluorine-18-fluoromisonidazole, that detect tumor hypoxia, which can affect tumor response to radiation therapy (Rajendran et al. 2006). The phe-

---

[1] Amino acids are the building blocks of proteins.

[2] In medicine, hypoxia refers to a shortage of oxygen in the body.

[3] In chemistry, an analog refers to a substance which is similar in structure to another substance.

nomenon that cells are more sensitive to radiation in the presence of oxygen is well-established (Mottram 1936), and resistance to radiation has been observed in some tumors with considerable hypoxic fractions. Radiolabeled peptides, antibody fragments, and, more recently, nanoparticles targeting different cell surface molecules also hold promise for tumor imaging and for targeted radionuclide therapy. Several of these radiolabeled peptides and antibody fragments targeting a variety of cell surface molecules have entered clinical trials (Sharkey and Goldenberg 2005).

These emerging radiotracer approaches hold promise for further individualization of cancer treatment. They will allow for the imaging of biological processes that are characteristic of cancer cells. For example, a variety of new anti-cancer drugs such as inhibitors of epithelial growth factor receptors have been found highly effective for killing cancer cells (Sequist et al. 2007). If additional tumor characteristics can be identified with target-specific molecular probes, it will become possible to select specific treatment strategies for individual patients and improve the probability of treatment success.

In addition, hybrid imaging devices, such as PET/CT, which combines the functional information provided by PET with the anatomic information provided by CT, have transformed staging and restaging of patients with cancer. As noted earlier, PET has the ability to detect differences in metabolic activity. However, without the map of the body that is provided by conventional imaging methods, it is difficult to pinpoint the organ or organ region in which abnormal activity is occurring. The diagnostic accuracy of PET/CT imaging with FDG exceeds that of PET or CT alone (Lardinois et al. 2003). Figure 3.2 depicts images taken with PET/CT in a patient with lung cancer. PET/magnetic resonance imaging (MRI), another hybrid imaging modality that merges anatomical and functional information, is currently under development (Cherry 2006). Although its role in patient care needs to be determined, it holds particular promise for studies of the brain.

3.2.2 Cardiovascular Disease

In cardiology, nuclear medicine imaging has assumed an important role in the diagnosis as well as the management of patients with coronary artery disease.[4] Myocardial perfusion imaging (Sidebar 3.2) is the most widely used approach in patients with suspected cardiac disease. Perfusion imaging of the heart is highly accurate for detecting the presence of coronary

---

[4]Coronary artery disease is caused by inadequate blood supply to the heart. This is generally caused by the narrowing or partially blockage of the arteries. Undetected or untreated coronary artery disease can lead to serious complications, such as a heart attack.

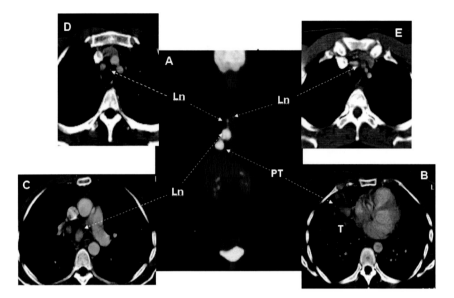

FIGURE 3.2 Staging of lung cancer with FDG and PET/CT. The whole-body image (Panel A) shows normal FDG uptake in the brain and the urinary bladder. In addition, several regions of intensely increased FDG uptake are seen in the chest. On the cross-sectional images of chest (Panels B through E), the primary tumor (PT, Panel B) is seen in the right lung (Ln) (arrow) with several malignant lymph nodes on the same side. There are additional malignant lymph nodes on the opposite side of the patient's chest (Panel E, arrows). SOURCE: Courtesy of Wolfgang Weber, University of California at Los Angeles (UCLA).

artery disease. In addition, the test can predict a patient's risk for further cardiac disease (e.g., non-fatal heart attack) and cardiac death. This allows physicians to provide better care to patients with advanced and disabling cardiac disease by guiding therapeutic decisions; the therapies can range from conservative, drug-based management of disease to more aggressive forms of intervention, such as surgery to restore blood flow. Because of the high prevalence of coronary artery disease, myocardial perfusion imaging studies have become the most widely used nuclear medicine imaging test. More than 7 million myocardial perfusion imaging studies are performed each year in the United States alone (Heinz Schelbert, UCLA, personal communication, March 8, 2007).

Approaches that primarily employ PET have been useful in delineating patterns of metabolism of both the healthy and the diseased heart. Metabolic activity demonstrated with PET and FDG in myocardial regions with diminished blood flow predicts an improvement in contractile function if

SIDEBAR 3.2 Myocardial Perfusion Imaging

Myocardial perfusion imaging is a test that allows doctors to examine blood flow to the heart muscle (i.e., myocardium). The patient is first injected with material labeled with a radionuclide, such as technetium-99m, thallium-201, or rubidium-82, which accumulates in the myocardium. Although a SPECT camera is more commonly used to take pictures of the heart, PET can also be used (Figure 1). Figure 2 depicts areas in the heart where there is abnormal blood flow.

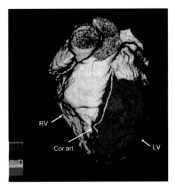

FIGURE 1 Fusion image of the heart's anatomy and blood flow. A three-dimensional fusion image of CT angiography and PET myocardial perfusion imaging is shown. The anatomy of the heart is shown in grey; the arrows indicate the left and right ventricles and the coronary arteries. The normal distribution of myocardial blood flow in the left ventricular myocardium is displayed in red. SOURCE:Reprinted by permission of the Society of Nuclear Medicine from Namdar et al. 2005.

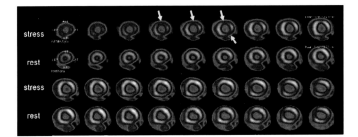

FIGURE 2 PET images of myocardial blood flow during stress and rest in a patient with coronary artery disease. Contiguous tomographic slices of the radiotracer uptake in the myocardium are shown (from left to right). Images in the upper row were obtained during stress and images at the bottom were obtained at rest. Light pink indicates normal and dark blue diminished blood flow. Note the area of reduced blood flow on the stress images (arrows) which is no longer seen on the rest images, indicating the presence of coronary artery disease. SOURCE: Courtesy of Marcelo Di Carli, Harvard University.

blood flow is restored by coronary artery revascularization (Tillisch et al. 1986). Furthermore, radiotracers of fuel substrates of the heart, such as carbon-11-labeled fatty acid, glucose, and acetate, that can be imaged with PET offer a means for identifying changes in the heart's substrate metabolism that are associated with age, obesity, or diabetes (Davila-Roman et al. 2002, Kates et al. 2003). Better understanding of these metabolic changes provides a framework for developing therapeutic strategies that may delay or avert progressive deterioration of heart muscle function and possible heart failure. Existing imaging techniques also offer a means for assessing the effectiveness of gene- and cell-based approaches for repairing the injured heart muscle tissue or for improving cardiac function. Changes in blood flow in response to angiogenic gene therapy with vascular endothelial growth factor, for example, can be monitored non-invasively (Udelson and Spiegler 2001). Similarly, effects of stem cell transplants on blood flow and metabolism on ischemically injured myocardium (i.e., after an acute myocardial infarction) can be demonstrated (Dobert et al. 2004). Nuclear medicine imaging will likely play an important role in the development and design of new therapies for cardiac disease.

New radiotracer techniques that are currently being investigated hold promise for the early diagnosis of coronary atherosclerosis.[5] Inflammation of lipid-rich deposits in the wall of the major arteries, called atherosclerotic plaques, can rupture and cause non-fatal heart attacks or cardiac death. Currently, blood biomarkers, such as C-reactive protein, that measure acute inflammation, have been associated with future coronary events; however, they do not indicate where the atherosclerotic plaque is located. The ability to pinpoint the locations of plaques within the coronary arteries may help predict which individuals are predisposed to serious cardiac events. Cardiovascular imaging with tomographic modalities such as CT is expected to help identify patients with vulnerable plaques earlier than with conventional coronary angiography (Schoenhagen et al. 2004). Nuclear medicine imaging studies have also indicated that localization may indeed be possible (Dunphy et al. 2005). For example, in patients at risk for stroke, FDG uptake was found to be considerably increased in diseased carotid arteries, reflecting severe inflammation of atherosclerotic lesions with a high potential of plaque rupture (Tawakol et al. 2006).

In patients with cardiovascular disease, hybrid imaging techniques such as PET/CT, SPECT/CT, and PET/MRI will likely facilitate the assessment of functional consequences of disease-related structural alterations. Conversely, they will also allow molecular and cellular processes to be assessed in absolute units and assigned accurately to structural alterations. These

---

[5]Atherosclerosis is a disease of the arteries in which fatty material builds up. The buildup is called plaque.

advantages offer opportunities for improving disease detection, character-ization, and treatment, as well as treatment monitoring in patients with cardiovascular disease. Their benefits could include more comprehensive assessments of cardiovascular health and disease and improved targeting of coronary vascular interventions, as well as accurate measurement of the severity of atherosclerotic disease, atherosclerotic plaques, and the effective-ness of plaque stabilizing therapies (Tarahan et al. 2006).

3.2.3 Neurological Disorders

A third clinical specialty where nuclear medicine imaging has played an important role in patient care is neurology. Radiotracer approaches aid in brain tumor evaluation and early identification of recurrence, in the planning of surgical treatment of seizure disorders, and, importantly, in assessing neurodegenerative disorders. As in other tumors, FDG is used in the diagnosis and characterization of brain tumors.

However, as noted earlier, the diagnostic accuracy with FDG has re-mained limited due to the high rate of glucose metabolism, and the high radiotracer uptake in normal brain tissue. This limitation has prompted the development and application of radiotracers such as carbon-11 methyl-methionine, fluorine-18-fluoro-l-phenylalanine, or fluorine-18-fluoro-L-thy-midine, which serve as markers of amino acid transport and metabolism and DNA synthesis. These radiotracers target tumor tissue in the brain and contribute to the grading of tumor aggressiveness and, more importantly, to distinguishing tumor recurrence from post-surgical tissue reactions and scar tissue formation (Chen et al. 2005, P. Chen et al. 2006) (Figure 3.3).

In seizure disorders, PET imaging with FDG has been found useful for localizing potentially epileptogenic regions of the brain, and their spatial distribution and extent. Accurate identification of such aberrant brain tis-sue is critical for determining eligibility of patients for surgical treatment approaches designed to abolish seizure disorders that are inadequately con-trolled by medications. Neurodegenerative disorders, such as Alzheimer's (Figure 3.4), Pick's, and Huntington's diseases (Sidebar 3.3), are typically associated with decreased glucose metabolism in certain parts of the brain. Each of these disorders is associated with diminished metabolism in specific brain regions that are distinguishable by FDG-PET (Silverman et al. 2001). Serial brain imaging studies with FDG-PET also allows monitoring of the rate of disease progression (Alexander et al. 2002).

Clinically it is difficult to differentiate mild cognitive impairment that is the result of a neurodegenerative disorder from that which derives from non-neurodegenerative causes or normal aging. This has prompted research and development of novel radioligands for targeting β-amyloid in senile plaques and tau in neurofibrillary tangles as noninvasive neuropathologic

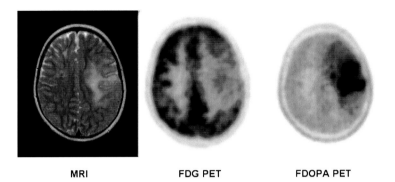

MRI   **FDG PET**   **FDOPA PET**

FIGURE 3.3 MRI and PET brain images in a patient with a brain tumor (grade II oligodendroglioma). The tumor in the left brain hemisphere as seen on the MRI image (left panel) is associated with diminished FDG uptake and thus reduced glucose utilization (center) but demonstrates intense amino acid uptake as seen on the FDOPA PET image (right panel). SOURCE: Courtesy of Wei Chen, UCLA.

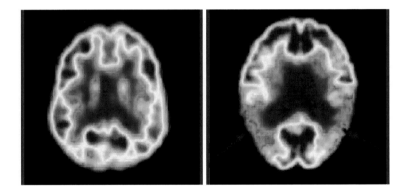

FIGURE 3.4 FDG-PET brain images in a normal volunteer (left panel) and in a patient with Alzheimer's disease (right panel). Tomographic slices through the brain at the level of inferior parietal/superior temporal cortex are shown. The color displayed in each part of the brain reflects the concentration of FDG corresponding to the metabolic activity of the neurons in that region. Red, orange, and yellow areas are (in decreasing order) the most active, while green, blue, and violet areas are progressively less active. Note that in neurologically healthy individuals, the entire cerebral cortex has a moderately high level of metabolism. In the patient with Alzheimer's disease, the arrows indicate areas of diminished metabolic activity in the patient's parietotemporal cortex, a region important for processing of language and associative memories. SOURCE: Courtesy of Daniel Silverman, UCLA.

SIDEBAR 3.3 Neurodegenerative Disorders

Alzheimer's disease is the most common form of dementia among elderly people, affecting an estimated 4.5 million Americans. It is a brain disorder that seriously affects a person's ability to carry out daily activities (NIA 2006). Its hallmark characteristics are the presence of excessive amyloid plaques (i.e., abnormal clumps) and neurofibrillary tangles (tangled bundles of fibers) that damage parts of the brain involved in thought, memory, and language (see Figure 3.5).

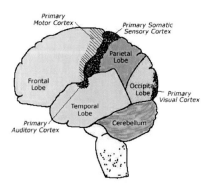

Brain diagram. SOURCE: http://www.aph.org/cvi/brain.html, adapted from Palmer (1999).

Huntington's disease is an inherited disease—that is, a mutation, or genetic change, in the Huntington's disease gene is passed on from a parent to a child. This change causes degeneration of brain cells that result in uncontrolled movement, loss of intellectual faculties, and emotional disturbances, such as mood swings and depression (NINDS 2006a).

Pick's disease is also known as fronto-temporal dementia. It is a syndrome associated with shrinking of the frontal and temporal anterior lobes of the brain (see diagram) that disrupts either an individual's ability to understand language (difficulty speaking or understanding speech) or causes changes in the person's behavior (e.g., loss of impulse control resulting in inappropriate social behavior, lack of empathy, apathy) (NINDS 2006b).

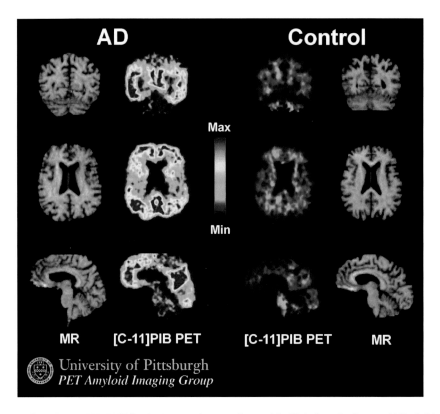

FIGURE 3.5 PIB PET brain images in a patient with Alzheimer's disease (AD, left) and in a normal control person. The PET PIB images are compared to anatomic maps of the brain generated with MRI which do not indicate any abnormalities. Note the intense radiotracer uptake in the AD patient (yellow and red colors) as compared to very little tracer uptake in the normal control (blue and purple). SOURCE: Courtesy of W. B. Klunk, University of Pittsburgh.

markers (Figure 3.5). Clinical studies support the promise of these novel radiotracers (e.g., the carbon-11-labeled Pittsburgh compound B (PIB) or the fluorine-18-labeled-2-dialkylamino-6-acylmalononitrile-substituted naphthalenes) for separating early stages of neurodegeneration from other age-related causes of cognitive impairment (Klunk et al. 2004). These radiotracers also appear to be useful for monitoring disease progression and outcomes of drug treatment (Engler et al. 2006).

Another important future goal will be to develop improved diagnostics and protective therapies for neurological disorders, such as Alzheimer's and Parkinson's diseases. To reach this goal, a more detailed understanding of the molecular changes that occur in the brain during the early stages of disease development will be required. Furthermore, increasing the availability of radiotracers that have been developed to pinpoint specific molecular changes and monitor response to therapy will enable us to reach this goal. For example, many radiotracers, such as fluorine-18-fluoroDOPA, for assessing the integrity of the brain dopamine system have been developed but are not readily available. Making these and other radiotracers more widely available could result in more accurate diagnosis and differential diagnoses of Parkinson's disease (Piccini and Whone 2004). In addition, other neurotransmitter systems (e.g., cholinergic, noradrenergic, serotonergic) also degenerate in Parkinson's disease, and the use of imaging to monitor changes in these systems, particularly in relation to disease progression, could represent another important future research direction (Brooks 2007).

Similarly, treating psychiatric disorders, such as depression, schizophrenia, and addiction, is a special challenge. Many of the existing treatments are inadequate, with major side effects or high non-response rates. In the future, the widespread availability of highly specific radiotracers that can be used in basic neuroscience research in humans can be expected to aid in understanding the biological processes of these diseases and, ultimately, the development of better treatments (Koob 2006, Zipursky et al. 2007).

3.2.4 Drug Development

In addition to its role in patient care, nuclear medicine imaging has the potential to accelerate the drug development process and substantially reduce the time and expense of bringing a drug to market. As described in Chapter 2, use of nuclear medicine imaging during the drug development process could identify which drugs should advance from animal to human studies, validate the mechanism of drug localization, evaluate drug distribution to target tissue, establish the drug occupancy of receptor sites, assess the actions of new agents on specific molecular targets or pathways, and determine appropriate dose range and regimen (Eckelman 2003).

Already, the pharmaceutical industry increasingly relies on small animal imaging laboratories for drug development and evaluation. Small animal imaging laboratories equipped with nuclear medicine imaging devices such as microPET or microSPECT but also with microCT, microMRI, and optical (e.g., bioluminescence and fluorescence) imaging systems offer an ideal environment for rapid and cost-efficient screening and development of new molecular probes and drugs. The new image-based assays account therefore for most of the newly developed radiopharmaceuticals in both academia and industry. Using small-animal imaging instruments and radiolabeled versions of drug candidates in which a carbon atom or other atoms of the drug molecule are substituted with a radionuclide of the same element, the binding of drug candidates to target and non-target tissues can be determined with relative ease and tissue pharmacokinetics can be studied. Furthermore, with targeted radiotracers, the efficiency of target occupancy and inhibition can be assessed non-invasively. Based on these animal data, imaging biomarkers can be developed to monitor treatment effects and to determine optimal drug doses on a molecular level in clinical studies. The small imaging devices also offer a means for rapid screening of potential drug candidates. For example, the effects of novel compounds on cell proliferation or cell metabolism can be determined in small-animal tumor models with fluorine-18-FLT and fluorine-18-FDG and thus serve as a "generic pharmacodynamic readout" (Leyton et al. 2005).

3.3 IMPEDIMENTS TO PROGRESS AND CURRENT AND FUTURE NEEDS

As described above, nuclear medicine imaging has the potential to further improve patient care in a variety of ways. However, the actual number of new radiotracers introduced into clinical practice over the past 10 years has been very limited. For example, although this chapter discusses a significant number of PET agents, only one agent (FDG) is used in more than 95 percent of all clinical PET studies. It is clear that the transfer of promising radiopharmaceutical and molecular probes from small animals to humans faces considerable hurdles. In part, this reflects the uncertain path that any drug must follow as it goes from discovery into application. For radiopharmaceuticals there are the added economic concerns of the relatively small market, even for common indications such as cancer. Some specific barriers are listed below.

1. **Regulatory Impediments.** Taken together, the regulatory impediments that limit approval and reimbursement for novel radiopharmaceuticals are the most important barrier to the continuing development and introduction of novel radiopharmaceuticals into clinical nuclear medicine practice. For example, the 1997 FDA Modernization Act, and the congressional and regulatory action that accompanied the enacting of this legislation, made possible the implementation of FDG-PET imaging as a clinical reality. A time table was proposed in the act, according to which more complete regulatory guidance should have been developed by the Food and Drug Administration (FDA) for facilitated regulation within 2 years. We are at the 10-year mark now, and no new regulation has yet been enacted to deal with the special features required for review and approval, or with clearance for reimbursement of novel nuclear medicine imaging procedures. This lack of clarity about process limits incentive to develop new agents and discourages commercial investment. It would be helpful if more spe-

cific guidance for diagnostic imaging drugs could be developed soon by the FDA.

The recent introduction of the exploratory investigational new drug (eIND) by the FDA will likely help in bringing new radiotracers into the human environment; the eIND limits the requirements for extensive toxicology testing, which, given the long history of safety of tracer procedures, may be excessive. Additional benefits would come from targeted support for phase 0 and phase I clinical trials of new agents within academic centers, which are still the most likely sites for development of new agents. The growing complexities of clinical regulations for early clinical trials for diagnostic imaging agents pose considerable financial burdens that are frequently beyond the means of investigators in academia. In the past, such costs were often defrayed by diversion of clinician income. However, with continued reductions in reimbursement, increased competition between imaging centers for patients, and increasing administrative and personnel costs, clinical practice resources have declined and are no longer sufficient to support initial clinical evaluation studies of new molecular probes.

The need for patient confidentiality and for protection and safety of human subjects is acknowledged by investigators, but regulatory and oversight requirements by institutional review boards[6] are, at times, excessive. Associated administrative burdens, together with excessive delays for institutional review and approval of study protocols have impeded clinical research. Stringent confidentiality requirements, such as those mandated by the Health Insurance Portability and Accountability Act,[7] pose additional difficulties (DHHS 2003). In many instances, these requirements have precluded long-term follow-up studies of patients, which are needed to assess the efficacy of new diagnostic approaches. There is growing concern that these regulatory hurdles have impeded translational research to the extent that some major clinical investigations have migrated from the United States to other countries with less stringent requirements.

2. Limited Radiotracer Availability and Distribution. Radiotracers for nuclear medicine imaging are supplied on a dose basis through networks of radiopharmacies and radiopharmaceutical distribution centers. Most radiopharmaceutical distribution centers in the United States are located within a less than 100-mile radius of nuclear medicine imaging facilities. This allows for a steady and reliable supply of radiotracers including those labeled with relatively short-lived positron emitting radionuclides such as fluorine-18-deoxyglucose (110-min physical half-life). Supply of

---

[6]Institutional review boards are internal groups who review and monitor biomedical research being conducted in human subjects at a given institution.

[7]The Health Insurance Portability and Accountability Act of 1996 mandated the adoption of Federal privacy protections for individually identifiable health information.

compounds labeled with radionuclides of shorter physical half-lives (e.g., 10 to 30 min) is, however, not possible through these distribution centers. Their use is therefore confined to institutions capable of onsite radionuclide production and radiotracer chemistry. Labeling of these radiotracers with longer lived radionuclides such as fluorine-18 will be important, because it will provide greater clinical availability and use. This impediment is further explored in Chapters 5 and 6.

   3.   Need for Standardization and Harmonization of Nuclear Imaging Procedures. Procedural aspects of nuclear medicine imaging vary, at times greatly, across institutions and thus may complicate or in some instances even preclude meaningful assessments of the clinical value and efficacy of nuclear medicine imaging. Examples of the characteristics that vary include the timing of image acquisition after radiotracer administration, data handling, and data storage. Accordingly, there is a need for greater uniformity of nuclear medicine imaging, including universally accepted image-derived measures of regional tissue function. Standardization of imaging study protocols, of image formatting, data handling, and data storage, as well as of image-derived parameters, will be especially critical for design and performance of multi-center clinical trials for drug evaluation and determination of efficacy of newly developed imaging approaches.

4

Targeted Radionuclide Therapy

Modern cancer therapy has proven partially successful in treating and prolonging the lives of patients with many common types of cancer. This limited success is due in part to the relative lack of specificity seen for many of the primary classes of anticancer agents and cytotoxic technologies in current medical practice. For most current cancer treatment options available today (e.g., conventional chemotherapy, external radiotherapy), the approach has been to destroy populations of cells that show uncontrolled growth. This focus on nonspecific cell division implies that the treatment will often be nonselective, damaging rapidly dividing nontumor cells, such as those in the gut. However, in recent years, there has been a much greater emphasis on "targeted therapies" that are designed to damage only the cancerous cells. There are currently hundreds of new pathway-targeted anticancer agents undergoing phase II and phase III clinical trials. Targeted radionuclide therapy is just one type within the category of "targeted therapies." At present, effective targeted radiopharmaceutical therapeutics have been developed and validated for a few tumor types, such as malignant lymphoma; for most other tumor types, the older nonspecific types of cancer treatments are still the dominant form of therapy.

This chapter describes the unique promise of targeted radionuclide therapy (Sidebar 2.2) and highlights what is needed to facilitate the translation of new targeted radionuclide therapies into clinical practice. To obtain information needed for this chapter, the committee consulted with leaders in the fields of radiation oncology, nuclear medicine, oncology, and chemistry from both industry and academia to identify the most critical needs for advancing targeted radionuclide therapy. The issues considered included the impact of deficiencies in radionuclide availability, trained personnel, and funding of the field.

The chapter is divided into the following sections:

- Background (4.1),
- Significant Discoveries (4.2),
- Current State of the Field and Emerging Priorities (4.3),
- Current Impediments (4.4),
- Recommendations (4.5), and
- Conclusions (4.6).

4.1 BACKGROUND

Radiation therapy uses ionizing radiation to kill cancer cells and shrink tumors by damaging the cells' DNA, thereby stopping these cells from continuing to grow and divide. The most common way of exposing cancer patients to radiation is through external radiation therapy. With this approach, only a limited area of the body is irradiated by delivering a beam of high-energy x rays to the main tumor. Targeted radionuclide therapy, on the other hand, is like chemotherapy, because it is a systemic treatment; it uses a molecule labeled with a radionuclide to deliver a toxic level of radiation to disease sites. Unlike tumor-directed drugs and toxins, which kill only the directly targeted cells, a unique feature of radionuclides is that they can exert a "bystander" or "crossfire" effect (Figure 4.1), potentially destroying adjacent tumor cells even if they lack the specific tumor-associated antigen or receptor. In addition, a systemically administered targeted radiotherapeutic that combines the specificity of cancer cell targeting with the known antitumor effects of ionizing radiation has the potential to simultaneously eliminate both a primary tumor site and cancer that has spread throughout the body, including malignant cell populations undetectable by diagnostic imaging. Figure 4.2 illustrates and contrasts the differences between direct and bystander killing of tumors.

In targeted radionuclide therapy, the biological effect is obtained by energy absorbed from the radiation emitted by the radionuclide. Whereas the radionuclides used for nuclear medicine imaging emit gamma rays, which can penetrate deeply into the body, the radionuclides used for targeted radionuclide therapy must emit radiation with a relatively short path length. There are three types of particulate radiation of consequence for targeted radionuclide therapy—beta particles, alpha particles,[1] and Auger

---

[1]An alpha particle is sub-atomic matter consisting of two protons and two neutrons.

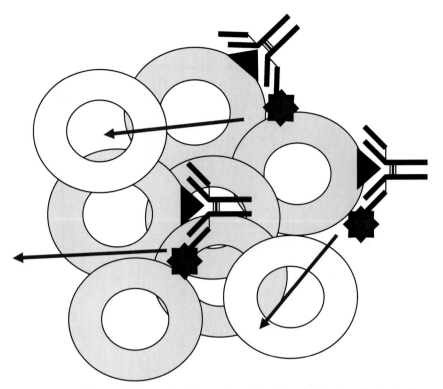

FIGURE 4.1 Schematic illustrating bystander effect for a labeled antibody (yellow circles = normal cells, light blue circles = tumor cells, the red triangles = antigen expressed on tumor cells, red Y-structure = antibody labeled with a radionuclide).

electrons[2]—which can irradiate tissue volumes with multicellular, cellular and subcellular dimensions (Figure 4.3), respectively. In some cases, mixed emitters are used to allow both imaging and therapy with the same radionuclide (e.g., the mixed beta/gamma emitter iodine-131). Moreover, within each of these categories, there are multiple radionuclides with a variety of tissue ranges, half-lives, and chemistries, offering the attractive possibility of tailor-making the properties of a targeted radionuclide therapeutic to the needs of an individual patient. The further development of this field is driven by the desire to move away from nonspecific toxic therapies commonly used in oncology and toward much less toxic targeted treatments, which impact only the targeted tissues.

---

[2]The second electron that is ejected after emission of an initial electron from an atom is known as an Auger electron.

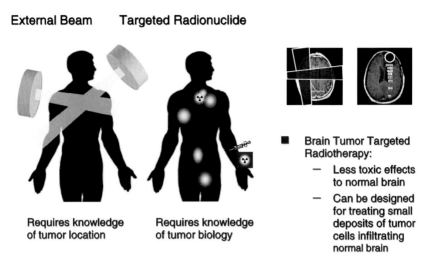

FIGURE 4.2 External beam therapy and targeted radionuclide therapy for the treatment of brain tumor. SOURCE: Courtesy of Michael Zalutsky, Duke University.

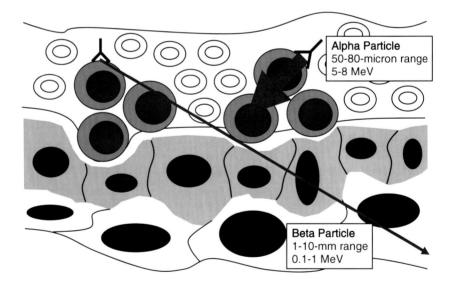

FIGURE 4.3 Penetrating power of alpha and beta particles. SOURCE: Courtesy of Joseph Jurcic, Memorial Sloan-Kettering Cancer Center.

SIDEBAR 4.1 Non-Hodgkin's Lymphoma

Lymphomas are a heterogeneous group of malignancies of the lymphatic system, which is a network of lymph vessels that is an integral part of the immune system. Other parts of the lymphatic system include the lymph nodes, tonsils, spleen, and thymus. Broadly, lymphomas are classified into two categories: Hodgkin's lymphoma (also known as Hodgkin's disease) and non-Hodgkin's lymphoma. Non-Hodgkin's lymphoma accounts for 85 percent of all lymphomas, and within this subgroup, there are many types of non-Hodgkin's lymphoma that can be classified by cell type (B-cell versus T-cell) or by level of aggressiveness.

At present, there are two commercially approved radioimmunotherapy agents, yttrium-90 ibritumomab tiuxetan (Zevalin®; Biogen-Idec Pharmaceuticals, San Diego, CA, approved by the Food and Drug Administration [FDA] in 2002) and iodine-131 tositumomab (BEXXAR®, GlaxoSmithKline, Philadelphia, PA, approved in 2003), both of which are used to treat indolent B-cell lymphoma (Sidebar 4.1) and related cancers. Both compounds target a B-cell[3] restricted lineage protein (i.e., CD20 surface antigen) expressed on B-cells, which is observed in more than 95 percent of patients with B-cell malignancies, and produce excellent clinical results: on the order of 60—80 percent overall response and 20—40 percent complete response rates[4] for patients with relapsed, recurrent, or refractory[5] indolent[6] B-cell lymphoma (Pohlman et al. 2006, Davies et al. 2004, Press 2003, Witzig et al. 2002). Although the radiobiologic principles and dosimetric requirements for the effective use of these two agents are still not fully understood, the clinical response shows that a single cycle of treatment with either of these two radiopharmaceuticals can result in essentially the same level of tumor response as multiple cycles of conventional chemotherapy, generally with a fraction of the toxicity (Macklis 2004).

In general, the use of both compounds involves a sequence of diagnostic and therapeutic sessions extending over about 7 to 10 days, where a com-

---

[3]B-cells are lymphocytes, or white blood cells, that are produced in the bone marrow and play an important role in immune response. B-cells make antibodies to help fight infection.

[4]Response rate is the percentage of patients who show a partial or complete response to a given treatment.

[5]In medicine, refractory disease refers to a condition that is unresponsive to treatment.

[6]Patients with indolent lymphoma generally have longer survival than patients who are diagnosed with high-grade lymphoma.

bination of medications is given and their biodistribution imaged. A patient treated with Zevalin® is first given a dose of nonradioactive antibody intravenously, followed by an infusion of a monoclonal antibody labeled with a gamma-emitting radionuclide (indium-111) as a tracer. The patient then undergoes an imaging study using a gamma camera (see Figure 4.4) that allows a physician to evaluate how the agent is distributed and cleared in the body. Finally, the patient is given a therapeutic dose of the monoclonal antibody radiolabeled with a beta-emitting radionuclide (yttrium-90) intravenously. Figure 4.5 illustrates how tumor response can be evaluated in a lymphoma patient treated with Zevalin® through the use of computed tomography (CT) and positron emission tomography (PET) scans.

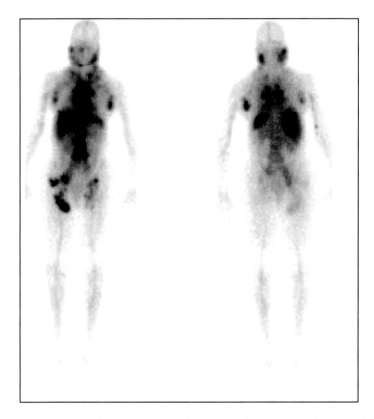

FIGURE 4.4 Initial radionuclide scan of patient infused with indium-111 labeled anti-CD20 antibody in preparation for a subsequent therapeutic infusion with an yttrium-90-labeled antibody (ibritumomab tiuxetan or Zevalin®) of the same specificity. SOURCE: Courtesy of Roger Macklis, Cleveland Clinic.

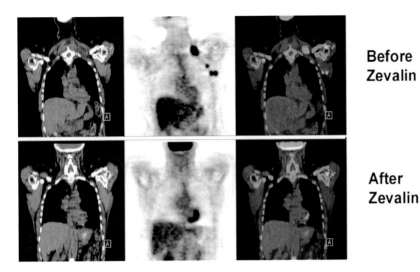

Before
Zevalin

After
Zevalin

FIGURE 4.5 This set of "before and after" PET/CT images demonstrates the use of these nuclear imaging modalities to evaluate the clinical effects of radioimmunotherapy using radiopharmaceutical compounds such as yttrium-90 ibritumomab tiuxetan (Zevalin®) in the treatment of malignant lymphoma. SOURCE: Courtesy of Peter Conti, University of Southern California.

4.2 SIGNIFICANT DISCOVERIES

A number of critical observations and discoveries have emerged based on previous funding from the National Institutes of Health (NIH) and the Department of Energy (DOE) that have set the stage for advances such as those described below.

Two FDA-approved Labeled Antibodies for the Treatment of Lymphoma

Zevalin® and BEXXAR® are now in general clinical use with impressive response rates and comparatively limited and reversible toxicity. Acknowledged lymphoma experts have noted that the anti-CD20 radioimmunotherapy compounds represent the most active single agents ever developed for the treatment of indolent B-cell lymphoma.

Other Antibodies and Radionuclides in Pre-Clinical and Early Clinical Phases of Testing

Many of these classes of biologically targeted radiopharmaceuticals have shown clear objective responses with acceptable toxicity levels (DeNardo

2005, Sharkey and Goldenberg 2005). These newer classes of therapeutic radiopharmaceuticals include compounds incorporating different antibodies, different radionuclides, and different modes of use. Several groups have recently published results of preclinical and early clinical studies using small molecules or antibodies directed against more common cancers (e.g., lung, breast, colorectal, and brain cancers) and have demonstrated proof of principle. These radioimmunotherapy agents undergoing preclinical and early clinical testing include a variety of radionuclides (with alpha, beta, gamma, and mixed emission spectra), linker chemistries, and half-lives.

Translation of Alpha Particle-Emitting Radiotherapeutics from the Laboratory to the Clinical Setting

Basic chemical advances in labeling molecules at high levels of radioactivity have led to the ability to assess the therapeutic potential of alpha-emitting radionuclides in preclinical models of human malignancy. The predicted localized cytotoxicity of alpha particles has been demonstrated, providing compelling evidence for initiating clinical trials with monoclonal antibodies radiolabeled with an alpha-emitting radionuclide in patients with leukemia and brain tumors.

Therapeutic Benefit in Minimum Residual Disease[7] Settings

Used in an adjuvant (i.e., postsurgical) setting, the clinical role of radioimmunotherapy would be to eradicate small nests of cells rather than large solid tumors for which much higher doses of radiation would be necessary.

4.3 CURRENT STATE OF THE FIELD AND EMERGING PRIORITIES

We are now entering an era of personalized medicine guided by new insights into basic biology and genetics that provide a better understanding of the steps that lead to cancer and other complex diseases. Medical practitioners now realize that tailoring treatment by taking into account an individual's anatomy, physiology, and genetic background is often required, not only for judicious selection of the drug to be administered but also for determining the appropriate dose of the pharmaceutical. For example,

---

[7]Minimal residual disease (MRD) is evidence for the presence of residual malignant cells at a subclinical level, when few or no cancer cells can be detected by conventional means. In a patient who has been treated, detection of MRD can indicate that treatment has not been curative. MRD can thus distinguish patients who need more intensive treatments from those who do not.

oncologists now are learning to use genetic signatures to determine which breast cancer patients might benefit most from various kinds of cytotoxic chemotherapy and which patients are not good candidates for standard treatments (O'Shaughnessy 2006).

Targeted radionuclide therapy has unique promise as a vehicle for personalized treatment of cancer, because both the targeting vehicle and the radionuclide can be tailored to the individual patient. Looking to the future, we can envision the following scenario:

- Treatment planning will be based on anatomic and molecular characteristics determined by imaging and complemented by genetic evaluation. High-resolution anatomic imaging will provide information on tumor size, location, and multiplicity to guide in the selection of the radionuclide. Molecular imaging will identify appropriate therapeutic targets that are overexpressed on the tumor cells.

- Sophisticated modeling and dosimetry software will be used to determine the best combination of radionuclide and targeting vehicle for attacking the tumor while avoiding harm to normal tissues. To ensure that all tumor cells are destroyed, it may be necessary to utilize "radiotherapeutic cocktails" formulated from radionuclides emitting different types of radiation, molecular carriers with different biological properties (antibodies, peptides, organic molecules) and binding to multiple tumor-associated targets. Monitoring of the distribution of the targeted radiotherapeutic agent or its surrogate by PET or single photon emission computed tomography will be done to plan subsequent dosing.

- Evaluation of tumor response by molecular imaging will allow the oncologist to evaluate response to treatment and tailor the next treatment to the altered status of the tumor cells (a process known as adaptive radiotherapy). For example, a patient initially treated with a targeted radiotherapeutic with a high-energy beta-emitting radionuclide that reduces tumor volume may subsequently be treated for residual disease with a targeted radiotherapeutic with an alpha-emitting radionuclide that has much more focal radiation (Figure 4.3). Moreover, postirradiation response could also alter receptor target populations on the tumor cells, which would require altering the molecule to which the radionuclide is attached. It is this flexibility that makes this approach to cancer treatment attractive.

Implicit in the above scenario is the availability of truly effective targeted radiotherapeutic agents for solid tumors, such as breast, colon, prostate, and lung cancers, that are less radiosensitive and less accessible than lymphomas, where targeted radionuclide therapy has already demonstrated meaningful results. A number of broad emerging research priorities, described in the following section, show promise for achieving this goal and are likely to have a considerable impact on targeted radionuclide therapy in the future.

4.3.1 Broad Emerging Research Priorities

The committee identified the following research priorities for targeted radionuclide therapy.

Optimal Radionuclides for Therapy

- **Alpha-Emitting Radionuclides.** The range of alpha particles in tissue is only a few cell diameters, offering the exciting prospect of matching the cell-specific nature of molecular targeting with radiation of a similar range of action. Another attractive feature of alpha particles for targeted radionuclide therapy is that, as a consequence of their high linear energy transfer, they have greater biological effectiveness than either conventional external beam x-ray radiation or beta emitters. Studies performed in cell culture have demonstrated that human cancer cells can be killed even after being hit by only a few alpha particles (Akabani et al. 2006) and that unlike other types of radiation, where oxygen is necessary for free radicals to be generated, efficient cancer cell elimination can be achieved even in an hypoxic environment. Although the conceptual advantages of alpha particles have been appreciated for more than 25 years, clinical investigation of these promising targeted radiotherapeutics has only just begun. Phase I clinical trials (Sidebar 2.6) have been performed with bismuth-213- and astatine-211-labeled monoclonal antibodies in patients with leukemia and brain tumors (Couturier et al. 2005), respectively, and radium-223 is being evaluated in breast and prostate cancer patients with bone metastases (Nilsson et al. 2005). Even though these trials have not all been carried out at optimized dose levels, encouraging responses have been observed in some patients, with acceptable levels of toxicity in normal tissues. An important aspect of these trials is the demonstration that targeted radionuclide therapy with alpha particle emitters is now clinically and scientifically feasible due to advances in radiochemistry, providing further impetus for more extensive investigation of this promising therapeutic approach in cancer patients.
- **Beta-Emitting Radionuclides.** Currently, the targeted radiotherapeutics approved by the FDA for human use are limited to four beta emitters: yttrium-90 and iodine-131, which are used in tandem with monoclonal antibodies to treat non-Hodgkin's lymphoma, and samarium-153-EDTMP (Quadramet®) and strontium-89-chloride for palliation of bone metastases. However, the scope of preclinical and clinical research in the therapy field is much broader, involving at least eight additional beta-emitting radionu-

clides: lutetium-177, holmium-166, rhenium-186, rhenium-188, copper-67, promethium-149, gold-199, and rhodium-105 (Zalutsky 2003).

- **Auger Electron-Emitting Radionuclides.** Auger electron emitters, such as bromine-77, indium-111, iodine-123, and iodine-125, are also being investigated. When used in concert with targeting vehicles that can localize these subcellular-range radiations in close proximity to cellular DNA, studies in cell culture have shown highly effective and specific tumor cell killing (Adelstein et al. 2003, P. Chen et al. 2006). The development of a matrix of targeted therapeutics offering multiple radionuclide—molecular carrier combinations can provide the tools to implement targeted radionuclide therapy regimens that are optimally tailored to the needs of individual patients.

Enhancing Target Concentration

The achievement of a therapeutically relevant level of radioactive drug in a tumor is critically dependent upon the concentration of the molecular target within the tumor. A number of strategies are being investigated for increasing the copy number and homogeneity of molecular targets on malignant cell populations (Mairs et al. 2000).

Management of Minimum Residual Disease

MRD settings can be difficult to treat by conventional means; however, targeted radionuclide therapy is likely to have an impact in treating MRD. Encouraging results from a phase II trial have been reported in the use of radiolabeled anti-carcinoembryonic antigen (CEA) antibody as an adjuvant in the treatment of colorectal cancer patients with liver metastases (Liersch et al. 2005), consistent with proof-of-principle studies in animal models (Koppe et al. 2006). These studies suggest that use of targeted radionuclide therapy as an adjuvant after surgical debulking could be a promising therapeutic strategy and provide evidence that targeted radionuclide therapy can be effective in solid tumors when applied in a setting of MRD. Follow-up studies are currently underway to investigate the clinical efficacy of the radiolabeled anti-CEA antibody.

Similarly, some encouraging results have been reported in the treatment of glioblastoma multiforme (GBM), a very aggressive type of brain tumor with poor prognosis. Conventional therapies such as chemotherapy and external beam radiation are largely ineffective because of dose-limiting toxicity to normal brain tissue. Because most GBM kill through local invasion and rarely metastasize outside the cranium, the clinical potential of loco-regionally applied targeted radionuclide therapy is being evaluated for the treatment of this malignancy. More than 300 patients have been treated worldwide with radiolabeled monoclonal antibodies injected directly into the resection cavity created after surgical removal of visible tumor. Encouraging responses have been observed in many patients, with median survivals of up to 90 weeks seen in GBM patients treated with iodine-131-labeled anti-tenascin monoclonal antibody 81C6 compared with approximately 1-year survival for conventional combined-modality treatments (Reardon et al. 2006); furthermore, the toxic effects on normal tissues were low. Similar proof-of-principle studies involving other regionally confined targets have also been published (Koppe et al. 2006). As these examples illustrate, the strength of targeted radionuclide therapy is its ability to seek out microscopic, even subclinical, cancers and selectively deliver curative doses of radiation, and this should be vigorously explored.

Radiolabeled Small Molecules

Radiolabeled monoclonal antibodies have been the most widely pursued approach to targeted radionuclide therapy; however, smaller molecular carriers, such as peptides that regulate the endocrine system, have been found to offer advantages for certain applications. The advantages of these smaller molecules include rapid accumulation in tumor and clearance from most normal tissues, which make them well-suited to use in tandem with some of the most promising radionuclides for targeted radionuclide therapy such as astatine-211 and rhenium-188, which have half lives of less than 24 hours. A number of regulatory peptides and their corresponding receptors that are overexpressed on certain types of tumors are being evaluated for possible application of targeted radionuclide therapy. For example, the most clinically advanced example of this strategy is targeting of the somatostatin receptor. Somatostatin, which is a peptide hormone that regulates the endocrine system and its corresponding receptor, has been studied for targeted radionuclide therapy of medullary thyroid carcinomas and neuroendocrine tumors (Kwekkeboom et al. 2005). Labeled peptides that bind specifically to other regulatory peptide receptors are also being investigated (Matthay et al. 2006). Penetration of these exciting concepts into the clinical domain has been much slower in the United States than in Europe.

Pre-Targeting Strategies

One of the challenges of targeted radiopharmaceutical development has been achieving a balance between maximizing the absolute amount of radionuclide that can be delivered to the tumor and meeting the requirement that the tumor-to-normal organ dose ratios be as high as possible. The problem is that large molecules such as antibodies provide the highest tumor accumulation, while smaller molecules such as peptides provide the highest tumor-to-normal organ dose ratios. An intriguing solution would be to break the treatment strategy into two steps, the first involving an unlabeled macromolecule followed later by administration of a radiolabeled small molecule that binds specifically to the protein. Exciting results utilizing bispecific antibodies have demonstrated proof-of-principle of this approach in animal models of human cancer, and early clinical trials are in progress (Goldenberg et al. 2006).

Radiobiological Factors

Conventional perspectives on the response of tissues to radiation may not adequately describe and predict the effects of targeted radiotherapeutics on tumor and normal tissues (Wiseman et al. 2003, Gokhale et al. 2005, Du et al. 2004). Because biologically targeted radiopharmaceutical therapy is generally characterized by low dose rates, the recently suggested hypersensitivity of mammalian cells to low dose radiation may play a role (Enns et al. 2004). The radiation-induced biological bystander effect (RIBBE) also could have a profound effect on targeted radionuclide therapy (Mothersill and Seymour 2004). In this process, cells not directly hit by radiation can be killed efficiently through an indirect but as yet unidentified mechanism. This is contrary to conventional radiation biological wisdom, which considers cell death to be a direct consequence of radiation traversal and energy deposition. These findings may have implications for targeted radionuclide therapy because if RIBBE could be harnessed, it could help compensate for variability in radiation dose deposition which is the bane of targeted radionuclide therapy (O'Donoghue et al. 2000). Although most work to date has been done with external beam radiation, investigations of low-dose hypersensitivity RIBBE with targeted radiopharmaceuticals are moving forward (Boyd et al. 2006) and could lead to novel strategies for cancer treatment. However, at present, both the radiobiology and the dosimetry of this field are topics of intense debate, and the implications for treatment are unclear.

4.3.2 Specific Research Priorities

For targeted radiopharmaceuticals to have a larger role in cancer treatment, the following key issues must be resolved:

• labeling methodologies that circumvent problems caused by high radiation levels (i.e., radiolysis) that are reliable for preparing clinical doses of therapeutic radiopharmaceuticals;
• more stable labeling methods for alpha emitters, particularly actinium-225 and astatine-211, to maximize the therapeutic potential of therapeutics labeled with these radionuclides;

- improvements in specific activity of labeled drugs to exploit highly tumor-specific but low-abundance molecular targets for cancer therapy;
- more universal methods for constructing targeted therapeutics that can be used with a variety of radionuclides;
- identification of a biomarker to predict normal organ response (includes effects of prior therapies);
- practical methods for calculating dose to tumor and normal tissues for radiation of short range and high potency (i.e., alpha particle and Auger electron emitters); and
- strategies for reducing toxic effects to the kidneys from promising radiotherapeutics of lower molecular weight.

4.4 CURRENT IMPEDIMENTS TO FULL IMPLEMENTATION OF TARGETED RADIOPHARMACEUTICAL THERAPEUTICS

The committee solicited input from individuals working in academia and in industry to identify current obstacles to the advancement of targeted radionuclide therapy. The following two major impediments were identified.

1. **Shortage of Radionuclides.** Many of the most important radionuclides that are needed for determination of patient-individualized dosimetry and pharmacokinetics[8] (iodine-124 and zirconium-89) or treatment (copper-67, bromine-77, and astatine-211) require production at an accelerator of higher energy and complexity than the small cyclotrons found in PET centers. The lack of a dedicated high-energy accelerator for the production of these and other radionuclides that form the basis for the future of targeted radionuclide therapy is a major barrier to progress in this field. Limitations in radionuclide availability restrict research and development in radiochemistry and radiobiology, assessment of efficacy, training, and clinical implementation. Of the five radionuclides identified as essential for therapeutic nuclear medicine (lutetium-177, astatine-211, yttrium-90, rhenium-186, and rhenium-188; see Chapter 5), only yttrium-90 is readily available in a form approved for use in humans. To allow individualized treatment, the armamentarium of radionuclides available in a form suitable for clinical use needs to be drastically increased.

2. **Cumbersome Regulatory Requirements.** There are three primary impediments to the efficient entry of promising new radiopharmaceutical compounds into clinical feasibility studies: (i) complex FDA toxicology and

---

[8]Pharmacokinetics is a branch of pharmacology that studies what the body does with a drug to which it is exposed to. (i.e., how it is absorbed, distributed, metabolized, and excreted).

other regulatory requirements (i.e., lack of regulatory pathways specifically for both diagnostic and therapeutic radiopharmaceuticals that take into account the unique properties of these agents); (ii) lack of specific guidelines from the FDA for good manufacturing practice of PET radiodiagnostics and other radiopharmaceuticals; and (iii) lack of a consensus for standardized image acquisition in nuclear medicine imaging procedures and protocols appropriate for multi-institutional clinical trials.

The costs associated with meeting the FDA toxicology requirements for evaluating a new radiotracer in humans are beyond the budgets of academic institutions and are a major regulatory impediment to radiopharmaceutical development and translation to clinical practice. Moreover, the level of evaluation required is beyond what is considered to be scientifically justified for a chemical compound typically administered once or twice at a tracer (i.e., not pharmacologically effective) level.[9]

4.5 RECOMMENDATIONS

RECOMMENDATION: *Clarify and simplify regulatory requirements, including those for (A) toxicology and (B) current good manufacturing practices (cGMP) facilities.*

Implementation Action A, Toxicology: The FDA should clarify and issue final guidelines for performing preinvestigational new drug evaluation for radiopharmaceuticals, particularly with regard to the recently added requirement for studies to determine late radiation effects for targeted radiotherapeutics.

Implementation Action B, cGMP: The FDA should issue final guidelines on cGMP for radiopharmaceuticals. These guidelines should be graded commensurate with the properties, applications, and potential risks of the radiopharmaceuticals. Instead of regulating minimal-risk compounds with the same degree of stringency as de novo compounds and new drugs that have pharmacologic effects.

Implementation Action C: To develop prototypes of standardized imaging protocols for multi-institutional clinical trials, members of the imaging community should meet with representatives of federal agen-

---

[9]A therapeutic is designed to deliver a higher radiation dose than a diagnostic because its purpose is to kill cancer cells. Thus, the toxicology requirements are more stringent than those required for a diagnostic because of the need to ensure that tumor irradiation does not also result in excessive damage to normal tissues.

cies (e.g., DOE, NIH, FDA) to discuss standardization, validation, and pathways for establishing surrogate markers of clinical response.

4.6 CONCLUSIONS

As noted earlier, targeted radionuclide therapy has the promise to personalize treatment by tailoring the properties of the radionuclide and the targeting vehicle for each patient. BEXXAR® and Zevalin® demonstrate robust proof of principle that adding a radionuclide enhances the clinical efficacy when compared with treating the patient with the biologic agent (e.g., cold antibody) alone. In addition, targeted radiotherapeutics have the potential for treating patients at a lower cost and with less morbidity than more standard treatment procedures. For example, radiation synovectomy is an alternative to surgery for the treatment of rheumatoid arthritis that costs less and allows patients to return to normal life sooner. It is a relatively simple procedure that can be performed on an outpatient basis and that is under ongoing investigation in Europe, although the approach is relatively dormant in the United States.

Recent experience in Europe demonstrates the appeal of targeted radionuclide therapy to patients. Patients increasingly go to Europe to receive targeted radionuclide therapy treatments that are not available domestically, and the gap in technology is increasing. The French are constructing a consortium-funded, high-yield, and versatile cyclotron for radionuclide production that will become operational in 2008. Such a machine has been under discussion for more than 10 years in the United States, and if anything, we are further away than we were a decade ago from constructing this critical piece of infrastructure. For the United States to retain its status as a leader in the field, these hurdles will need to be addressed.

5

Availability of Radionuclides for Nuclear Medicine Research

This chapter addresses part of the fourth charge of the statement of task. It examines whether a shortage of radionuclides for nuclear medicine research exists, and if so, what impact it is having on basic and translational research, drug discovery, and patient care, and what short- and long-term strategies can be implemented to alleviate such shortages. The chapter is divided into the following sections:

- Background (5.1),
- Current State of Radionuclide Availability in the United States (5.2),
- Significant Discoveries (5.3),
- Current and Future Needs and Impediments (5.4), and
- Recommendations (5.5).

5.1 BACKGROUND

At the very heart of all nuclear medicine procedures is the need for year-round, reliable availability of radionuclides. Currently, more than 70 percent of all procedures in nuclear medicine are based on technetium-99m (Nuclear Energy Agency 2000), a radionuclide produced by individual generators that use material produced in reactors outside of the United States.[1] Growing use of positron emission tomography (PET) and targeted

---

[1]The availability of technetium-99m is currently being reviewed under the auspices of a separate National Research Council study and is beyond the scope of this report.

75

radionuclide therapy has created the need for steady supplies of a variety of other radionuclides, and the demand is expected to increase (Wagner et al. 1999).

The production of radionuclides in the United States can be traced to the graphite reactor at Oak Ridge National Laboratory (ORNL) shortly after World War II. In its first year of operation, hundreds of shipments of 60 different radionuclides were made. Production of radionuclides for biomedical research continued until the reactor was shut down in 1963. Based on the successes achieved and the interest created by this early work, radionuclides were produced throughout the 1960s and 1970s at universities and national laboratories that had reactors, cyclotrons, or other acccl-erators available (Sidebar 5.1).

Commercial producers and distributors have played an important role in supplying radionuclides such as molybdenum-99/technetium-99m, thal-lium-201, gallium-67, indium-111, and iodine-123. With the advent of PET technology, beginning in the late 1970s, the need for a more reliable supply of radionuclides with short half-lives drove industry to develop small cyclotrons for supplying the primary radiopharmaceutical, fluorine-18-fluorodeoxyglucose (FDG). However, the market for radionuclides such as copper-67 and astatine-211 has never been large enough to encourage in-dustry to produce them,[2] and they are not readily available from low-energy PET cyclotrons. The issue of such "exotic" radionuclides, or radionuclides requested by a fairly small number of investigators for their research stud-ies, has plagued the field for years. Many of these radionuclides will never be in high demand but could be important for advancing the understand-ing of fundamental biology or therapeutic efficacy (e.g., bromine-76 and copper-67).

5.2 SIGNIFICANT DISCOVERIES

Many of the discoveries associated with radionuclides were made pos-sible by government research funding, particularly DOE research fund-ing. The following examples indicate the variety and complexity of the types of investigations and discoveries that were made possible by these investments:

Molybdenum-99/Technetium-99m Generator

As mentioned earlier, technetium-99m is the most widely used radio-nuclide for nuclear medicine procedures in the world, accounting for more than 70 percent of all nuclear medicine procedures (Nuclear Energy Agency

---

[2]A list of commercially available radiopharmaceuticals is provided in Appendix C.

2000). The molybdenum-99/technetium-99m generator was invented at Brookhaven National Laboratory (BNL). This generator system is popular because the parent radionuclide (molybdenum-99) has a half-life of 66 hours while its decay product (technetium-99m) has a half-life of 6 hours. The differences in the half-lives and chemical properties of molybdenum and technetium are exploited to separate them in the generator (Sidebar 5.2). This separation can be repeated many times, and this system provides a nearly continuous supply of radionuclides at a low cost. Major efforts have been expended on developing the chemistry to incorporate technetium-99m into useful biological molecules. The results have included radiopharmaceuticals that assess cardiac function, blood flow, and bone metastases.

Carbon-11 Hot Atom Chemistry

The work of Alfred Wolf and co-workers throughout the 1960s and early 1970s at BNL laid the foundation for the production and labeling of carbon-11 in a variety of biologically active molecules. As shown in Sidebar 5.1, a carbon-11 atom produced in a particle accelerator will have a large amount of kinetic energy, more than enough to break ordinary chemical bonds. These particles are called *hot atoms*. Most of the science of radiotracers/radiopharmaceuticals, including radionuclide therapy, has its roots in hot atom chemistry.

Production Excitation Functions[3] for Fluorine-18, Carbon-11, and Oxygen-15

At the very heart of radiotracer research is the ability to produce sufficient quantities of radionuclide to be incorporated into biologically useful molecules. During the late 1970s, a group of researchers under the guidance of Alfred Wolf at BNL examined a number of excitation functions to demonstrate that a simple, low-energy, proton-only accelerator could produce the requisite quantities of the most widely used radionuclides for PET. This work encouraged a commercial company to design and build a small cyclotron dedicated to providing large quantities of fluorine-18, carbon-11, and oxygen-15 to PET centers. There are now nearly 200 of these cyclotrons positioned around the world providing an infrastructure for supply of FDG and other PET tracers (see Figure 6.1 for the geographic distribution of cyclotrons in the United States).

---

[3] The amount of radionuclide that is produced depends on the energy of the particle that is used to bombard the target. The yield of the radioactive product versus particle energy is called the excitation function.

SIDEBAR 5.1 Types of Machines that Produce Radionuclides and How Radionuclides Are Created

There are two main ways[a] of producing radionuclides with a nuclear reactor or with a particle accelerator. The two methods are complementary in providing a wide variety of radionuclides for research and patient care.

A nuclear reactor is a device in which nuclear chain reactions are initiated, controlled, and sustained at a steady rate. Nuclear reactors are most commonly used to generate electricity, but are also used as a neutron source to produce radionuclides (Figure 1).

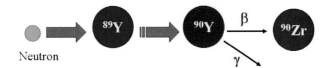

Neutron

FIGURE 1 Schematic of yttrium-90 (Y-90) generation via neutron capture of the stable element yttrium-89 (Y-89). Yttrium-90 is a radionuclide used in targeted radionuclide therapy which decays with a half-life of 2.7 days (see Chapter 7). SOURCE: Courtesy of Thomas Ruth, TRIUMF.

A particle accelerator is a device that uses electric fields to propel electrically charged particles to high speeds, which then collide with targets. Out of this collision, many subatomic particles are produced (http://www2.slac.stanford.edu/wc/ accelerator.html). Particle accelerators can be found in everyday use (e.g., the cathode ray in a television set), but are also used in other settings, such as to produce medical or research radionuclides (Figure 2). Broadly, there are two types of accelerators: linear (linac) and circular (cyclotron) (Figure 3). In a linear accelerator, particles are accelerated in a straight line, whereas in a circular accelerator, the particles move in a circular path.

---

[a]Another method that is used for radionuclide production involves the separation of fission products of uranium-235, which is used as the fuel in most nuclear reactors. This production method is currently used to produce molybdenum-99 for use in technetium-99m generators.

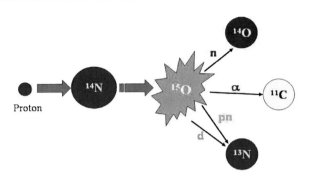

FIGURE 2 In radionuclide production, one element is transmuted into another. The above schematic illustrates how an atom of nitrogen is bombarded by a proton producing an excited oxygen atom (O-15) which then can emit any one of several particles to leave the new atom. In this case the new atoms are all positron-emitting radionuclides. These radionuclides can be separated by physical and/or chemical means. SOURCE: Courtesy of Thomas Ruth, TRIUMF.

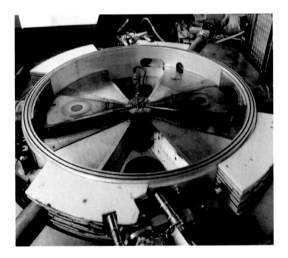

FIGURE 3 Photograph of the interior of a cyclotron shows the copper dees, the accelerating component of a cyclotron and the 4 "hills" of the magnet. This cavity is enclosed with a plate so that a chamber capable of sustaining a vacuum is formed. Ions of a light particle such as hydrogen or helium are injected into the center of the cyclotron where they are accelerated by the electrically charged dees. The dees are high-voltage cavities that change polarity (electrical charge) at a high frequency (radiofrequency = tens of megahertz). The magnet forces the charged particles to move in a circular path. As the particle gains energy the circular path increases in radius until it reaches the energy desired, whereupon it is extracted and directed to a target material where a nuclear reaction forms the radionuclide of choice (see Figure 1). SOURCE: Courtesy of Thomas Ruth, TRIUMF.

SIDEBAR 5.2 Generators

A generator is a device that is used to extract one nuclide from another. For example, technetium-99m is recovered from technetium generators, which are shielded cartridges that contain molybdenum-99. Saline solutions can be passed through these generators (a process known as "milking") to recover the technetium-99m.

Development of Practical Generator Systems

The ability to access PET radionuclides without the use of onsite accelerators or reactors depends upon the availability of generator-produced radionuclides. Lawrence Berkeley National Laboratory developed the first practical generators for the germanium-68/gallium-68 and the strontium-82/rubidium-82 pairs. Strontium-82 is now being used with increasing frequency for clinical cardiac studies. It is presently supplied through a consortium of accelerators throughout the world that run parasitically and is not under the control of the user community. With the increasing demand for the strontium-82 generator, the current sources may not be sufficient in sustaining availability of this radionuclide.

Production of Tungsten-188/Rhenium-188 Generator

ORNL developed the tungsten-188/carrier-free rhenium-188 perrhenic acid generator system. Rhenium isotopes have chemistry similar to that of technetium and thus are of interest for adapting the extensive labeling tools created for technetium-99m. Rhenium-188 in particular is attractive for certain therapy applications because it emits a high-energy beta particle and has a relatively short half-life.

5.3 CURRENT STATE OF RADIONUCLIDE AVAILABILITY IN THE UNITED STATES

The Department of Energy's (DOE) national laboratories remain the primary source of less commonly used or exotic radionuclides, produced from their large reactor and accelerator facilities. These facilities include the High Flux Isotope Reactor (HFIR) at ORNL, Brookhaven Linac Isotope Producer (BLIP) at BNL, the Isotope Production Facility at Los Alamos Nuclear Science Center (LANSCE) at Los Alamos National Laboratory

(LANL), and the Advanced Test Reactor (ATR)[4] at Idaho National Laboratory (INL). The facilities at the national laboratories were designed and operated to fulfill their missions in physics, materials science, and other research programs. In addition to performing their primary missions, these reactors and accelerators were made available for the production of radionuclides to be carried out in parasitic mode (i.e., while accelerators are in operation for other purposes). However, as the interest in exotic radionuclides has grown, the national laboratories have not been able to meet the demands of the research community for regular and continuous availability of these radionuclides. Not only have the operating schedules been dictated by the primary users, but radionuclide production has been limited by age-related degradation of the facilities and extended shutdowns for facility maintenance. Of the major operational facilities that support radionuclide production, HFIR at ORNL was first operated in 1965, ATR at INL in 1970, the ORNL calutrons in 1944, BLIP at BNL in 1972, and LANSCE at LANL in 1974. There are currently no plans to replace these facilities.[5]

Medium-sized research reactors located on university campuses have also complemented the large DOE facilities by providing research quantities of medical isotopes. One successful example is the radiochemical and radiopharmaceutical research, production, and education program at the Missouri University Research Reactor (MURR). MURR was evaluated and identified as the best program in the United States by the Nuclear Energy Research Advisory Committee (NERAC) subcommittee (Reba et al. 2000), and the National Radionuclide Production Enhancement Program recently recommended that the MURR receive federal support of $7 million to upgrade its facility to increase the quality and quantity of radionuclide production for research and clinical applications (SNM 2005). However, the number of university research reactors in the United States has been in steady decline since the early 1970s. Of the 25 university research reactors currently in operation, 11 are licensed at or higher than 1 MW; the other 14 reactors are low-power reactors suitable only for training purposes (Bernard and Hu 2000, Rogers 2002). Most of these reactors were built in the late 1950s or 1960s and require continued facility upgrades and maintenance in order to fulfill their missions in research and education. Table 5.1 lists the reactor and accelerator facilities in the United States that have medical radionuclide production capability.

---

[4]Although the ATR at INL is the largest research reactor in the United States, it is not designed to produce medical isotopes with short half-lives. There is, however, a plan by the state of Idaho to invest $2 million to upgrade its production capabilities that will enable medical isotope production by 2008 (Press Release, Dec., 29, 2006). More specifically, the funding allows for the installation of a Transfer Shuttle Irradiation Facility that will produce medical and other isotopes.

[5]There is a plan to invest $200 million to upgrade LANSCE.

TABLE 5.1 Reactor and Accelerator Facilities in the United States with Medical Radionuclide Production Capability

Location	Facility	Power	Medical Radionuclides Currently Produced
Reactors			
ORNL	HFIR	85 MW	^{225}Ac, ^{252}Cf, ^{43}K, ^{103}Pd, ^{188}W, ^{117m}Sn, ^{147}Pm, ^{177}Lu, ^{186}Re, ^{166}Ho, ^{194}Ir, ^{191m}Ir, and others
University of Missouri	MURR[a]	10 MW	^{32}P, ^{166}Ho, ^{192}Ir, ^{35}S, ^{186}Re, ^{90}Y, ^{51}Cr, ^{103}Pd, ^{177m}Lu, and others
Massachusetts Institute of Technology	MITR-II[a]	5 MW	^{198}Au, ^{90}Y, ^{192}Ir, and others (research quantities)
University of California at Davis	MNRC[a]	2 MW	^{125}I and others (research quantities)
Oregon State	OSTR[a]	1 MW	Variety (research quantities)
Accelerators			
LANL	LANSCE	800 MeV proton	^{26}Al, ^{67}Cu, ^{68}Ge, ^{82}Sr, ^{86}Y, ^{124}I, and others
BNL	BLIP	200 MeV proton	^{67}Cu, ^{82}Sr, ^{68}Ge, and others
Washington University	cyclotrons		^{64}Cu, ^{77}Br, ^{66}Ga, ^{124}I, ^{94m}Tc
Trace Life Sciences[b]	Various LINAC and cyclotrons		^{64}Cu, ^{67}Cu, ^{111}In, ^{123}I, ^{201}Tl

[a]Non-DOE facilities: University research reactors.
[b]Commercial production facility.

SOURCE: DOE Isotope Program.

Compounding these infrastructure issues is concern about the availability of enriched stable isotopes[6] that are used as target materials for the production of radionuclides, regardless of method. Nearly all enriched stable isotopes that are used in nuclear medicine are imported from foreign suppliers. The primary domestic source, calutrons[7] at ORNL, has been on standby

---

[6] Enriched stable isotopes refers to increasing the abundance of a particular isotope to levels above the naturally occurring abundance.

[7] Calutrons are devices used to increase the isotopic composition for an element based on electromagnetic separation of molecules of different mass.

since 1998 because of competitive pricing from foreign suppliers (Reba et al. 2000). According to a report produced by the NERAC (Wagner et al. 1999), ORNL had a substantial inventory of enriched stable isotopes. Although the supply is not seen as disappearing in the near term, there is a concern that without a clear plan to address future needs, researchers both in the United States and worldwide will face a shortage of enriched stable isotopes.

Research radionuclide distribution has also been affected by the Energy and Water Development Appropriations Act of 1990 (Public Law 101-101), which requires the DOE to operate on a full cost recovery[8] model (Sidebar 5.3). A consequence of this law has been the competing demand between producing high-cost, non-commercial radionuclides for researchers and supplying high-volume, commercial-use radionuclides to the private sector. The requirement for full cost recovery has made access to novel radionuclides cost-prohibitive for the vast majority of laboratories and clinics and is one of the major impediments to progress in nuclear medicine research.

A number of studies by different organizations, including the Institute of Medicine, have investigated the isotope (i.e., radionuclides and stable isotopes) needs of the country (Sidebar 5.4 provides a list of references). All of these studies came to the same conclusion: a dedicated radionuclide production facility is urgently needed to foster and facilitate research and training in the use of radionuclides in the biosciences and to provide a domestic, year-round, continuous supply of radionuclides for nuclear medicine practice.

5.4 CURRENT AND FUTURE NEEDS

To determine the current and future radionuclide production needs for furthering nuclear medicine research, the committee solicited input from experts in the field. Table 5.2 is a list of the radionuclides most frequently described as being essential to nuclear medicine research. Several of these research radionuclides are not being produced in sufficient quantities to meet the research demand. The technical and nontechnical needs and impediments are summarized in Sections 5.4.1 and 5.4.2, respectively.

5.4.1 Technical Needs and Impediments

There is no domestic (i.e., U.S.) source for most of the medical radionuclides used in day-to-day nuclear medicine practice. Furthermore, the lack of dedicated domestic accelerator and reactor facilities for year-round production of medical radionuclides for research is limiting the develop-

---

[8] Full cost recovery means recovering or funding the full costs of a project or service, including overhead.

SIDEBAR 5.3 The Energy and Water Development Appropriations Act of 1990 (Public Law 101-101)

P.L. 101-101 is one of two major laws that provide the authority to regulate radionuclide production and distribution in the United States. Unlike the Atomic Energy Act of 1954, which was passed to promote the production of radionuclides for research, the intended goal of P.L. 101-101 was to provide an incentive for cost-effectiveness by bringing the management of radionuclide production and distribution under one roof. Appropriations to the program are mainly applied to the maintenance and upgrade of production facilities. Under the DOE's Isotope Program[a] radionuclides are sold to researchers at prices that recover the direct production cost, while commercial customers pay the full cost including allocated facility costs. Note that no provision for the production of radionuclides made exclusively for research was made (IOM 1995). The Isotope Program's resources in millions of dollars are depicted in the figure below.

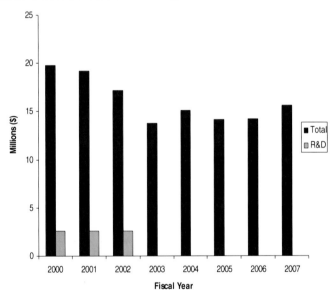

Annual Appropriations for the Department of Energy-Office of Nuclear Energy's (DOE-NE) Isotope Program, 2000-2006 ($ in millions) SOURCE: Data provided by DOE-NE.

---

[a]DOE's Isotope Program oversees the production and sales of radioactive and stable isotopes, along with related services, such as irradiation, target preparation and processing, and chemical separation.

**SIDEBAR 5.4 Studies Reviewing Isotope
Supply in the United States**

Separated Isotopes: Vital Tools for Science & Medicine, A Report of the National Research Council, National Academy Press, Washington, D.C., 1982. (NRC 1982)

Adelstein SJ, Manning JF, eds. Isotopes for Medicine & the Life Sciences. Committee on Biomedical Isotopes. Division of Health Sciences Policy, National Academy Press, Washington, D.C., 1995. (IOM 1995)

Ketchum LE, Green MA, Jurisson SS: Research Radionuclide Availability in North America. J. Nucl. Med. 38 (7): 15N-19N, and 38(8): 21N-48N, 1997. (Ketchum et al. 1997)

Medical Isotope Workshop, Spicer KM, Baron S, Frey GD, O'Brien H, Gostic RC, Rowe RW, Spellman RMN, eds: Med Coll of South Carolina, Pub, 1998. (Spicer et al. 1998)

Wagner HN Jr, Reba RC, Brown R, Coleman E, Knight L, Sullivan D, Caretta R, Babich JW, Carpenter A, Nichols D, Spicer K, Scott S, and Tenforde T. Expert Panel Forecast of Future Demand for Medical Isotopes. March, 1999, http://www.ne.doe.gov/nerac/isotopedemand.pdf (Wagner et al. 1999)

Reba RC, Atcher RW, Bennett RG, Finn RD, Knight LC, Kramer HH, Mtingwa S, Ruth TJ, Sullivan DC, and Woodward JB. Final Report, NERAC Subcommittee for Isotope Research & Production Planning. April 2000, pp 1-32. Published on line by DOE and viewed at http://www.nuclear.gov/nerac/finalisotopereport.pdf (Reba et al. 2000)

National Radionuclide Production Enhancement (NRPE) Program: Meeting Our Nation's Need for Radionuclides. Society of Nuclear Medicine. May 2005. (SNM 2005)

Audit Report: Management of the Department's Isotope Program. DOE/IG-0709. November 2005. (DOE 2005)

Rivard MJ, Bobek LM, Butler RA, Garland MA, Hill DJ, Krieger JK Muckerheide JB, Patton BD, Silberstein EB. The US national isotope program: Current status and strategy for future success. Applied Radiation and Isotopes 63 (2005) 157–178. (Rivard et al. 2005)

---

ment and evaluation of new radiopharmaceuticals. The parasitic use of physics machines has failed to meet the radionuclide type, quantity, timeliness of production, and cost requirements of the medical research community. For example, copper-67 has shown great promise as a therapeutic radionuclide, but it is available only through the parasitic use of accelerators with missions other than radionuclide production.[9] Another example is astatine-211, an alpha-emitting radionuclide that requires a medium-

---

[9] BNL, LANL, and Tri-University Meson Facility (TRIUMF) are only available for less than half of the year for radionuclide production.

TABLE 5.2 Therapeutic Radionuclides Used for Nuclear Medicine Research

Radionuclide	Description	Production
Lutetium-177	Beta emitter, 6.7-d half-life	Reactor
Astatine-211	Alpha emitter, 7.2-h half-life	Accelerator
Yttrium-90	Beta emitter, 64-h half-life	Reactor
Rhenium-186	Beta emitter, 3.7-d half-life	Reactor
Rhenium-188	Beta emitter, 17-h half-life	Reactor
Holmium-166	Beta emitter, 27-h half-life	Reactor
Iodine-131	Beta emitter, 8.0-d half-life	Reactor
Samarium-153	Beta emitter, 46-h half-life	Reactor
Bromine-77	Beta emitter, 57-h half-life	Accelerator
Copper-67	Beta emitter, 62-h half-life	Accelerator
Actinium-225	Alpha emitter, 10.0-d half-life	Accelerator
Strontium-89	Beta emitter, 50.5-d half-life	Reactor

energy alpha-particle accelerator for its production. There are only a few accelerators remaining in the United States that are capable of producing astatine-211 and these are primarily used for clinical PET programs and for radiation therapy.

Although procuring isotopes from foreign countries, such as Germany and Russia, and increasing international collaborations are worthwhile alternatives, relying solely on foreign sources has a number of drawbacks. These include increased transit time over international borders, which for radionuclides that decay during transport, is an important consideration; and possible changes in radionuclide production priorities that may adversely affect U.S. researchers. A number of studies that have reviewed this issue have concluded that the United States should have a dedicated radionuclide production facility to meet the needs of the research community (IOM 1995, Wagner et al. 1999, Reba et al. 2000). The operation of such a facility would have to be subsidized to allow researchers to explore new and novel uses of radionuclides.[10]

For research that uses short-lived radionuclides, it is essential to have an accelerator onsite to provide these radionuclides when needed. The

---

[10]The benefits of providing radionuclides at low cost are clear from the experience of Washington University, which received funding from the National Cancer Institute to produce nontraditional PET radionuclides, such as copper-64, gallium-66, bromine-76, and iodine-124, for users. Washington University has provided these nontraditional radionuclides on a low-cost (i.e., highly subsidized) basis to more than 30 research institutions that previously did not have the technical ability to produce them. By doing so, it has created a large enough demand to encourage commercial involvement. Today, copper-64 and iodine-124 are commercially available from MDS-Nordion and IBA Molecular, respectively.

existing hospital-based cyclotrons are, in general, fully committed to their own programs and cannot be considered as a reliable resource for exotic research radionuclides. In addition, many of these radionuclides can only be made on accelerators with energy of 30 MeV or above or require particles other than protons, neither of which can be provided by current hospital-based cyclotrons.

5.4.2 Non-Technical Needs and Impediments

The DOE-NE Isotope Program is failing to meet the needs of the research community because the effort is not adequately coordinated with NIH activities or with the DOE-Office of Biological and Environmental Research. Additionally, P. L. 101-101 (Sidebar 5.3), which requires full cost recovery for DOE-supplied radionuclides, whether for clinical use or research, has stifled research radionuclide production and radiopharmaceutical research. As a consequence, few new radiotracers have become commercially available over the past decade and there is a lack of radiotracers in the commercial pipeline.

In terms of research, the user community is a single investigator or small number of investigators, for whom the cost of producing exotic radionuclides exceeds available budgets. It has been difficult to include such expenses in research grants because the dollar value is disproportionately higher than other research expenses. Therefore, unlike commercial vendors who can pass on the costs to a wider user community, investigators looking into new ways to use radionuclides for diagnosis and treatment cannot afford the full costs of radionuclides sold by the DOE. Such a barrier reduces the demands for novel radionuclides. It has also created the perception that the nuclear medicine community is not interested because it is not requesting the radionuclides. While it is true that there are no new radionuclides with the requisite physical and chemical properties for use in imaging and therapy, there will continue to be investigations into new applications of the known radionuclides. Thus, an argument can be made that the DOE radionuclide production facility, which might benefit from new uses, should bear all or at least some of the development costs. However, the production facility is not a research organization, and so, some mechanism would need to be set up to vet applications for subsidy.

5.5 RECOMMENDATIONS

RECOMMENDATION 1: *Improve domestic medical radionuclide production. To alleviate the shortage of accelerator- and nuclear reactor-produced medical radionuclides needed for research, a dedicated accelerator and an upgrade to a nuclear reactor should be considered.*

This recommendation is consistent with other studies that have reviewed medical isotope supply in the United States and have come to the same conclusions (IOM 1995, Wagner et al. 1999, Reba et al. 2000).

RECOMMENDATION 2: *Review enriched stable isotope inventory and evaluate domestic supply options if needed. The current inventory of enriched stable isotopes is decreasing and there is growing concern that the aging calutrons cannot be operated cost-effectively to meet demand if reopened. The DOE should evaluate the option of a domestic enriched isotope supply source to ensure availability for medical research.*

6

Radiotracer and Radiopharmaceutical Chemistry

This chapter examines the "future needs for radiopharmaceutical development for the diagnosis and treatment of human disease," the "national impediments to the efficient entry of promising new radiopharmaceutical compounds into clinical feasibility studies and strategies to overcome them," and the "impacts of shortages of isotopes on nuclear medicine basic and translational research, drug discovery, and patient care, and short- and long-term strategies to alleviate these shortages if they exist" (charges 1, 3, and part of charge 4 of the statement of task). The content of this chapter, particularly the sections delineating needs and impediments, is derived largely from discussions with and presentations from chemists and other researchers working in the nuclear medicine field. The impact of the shortage of radionuclides was discussed in detail in Chapter 5.

The chapter is divided into the following sections:

- Background (6.1),
- Significant Discoveries (6.2),
- Current State of the Field and Emerging Priorities (6.3),
- Current Needs and Impediments (6.4), and
- Recommendations (6.5).

6.1 BACKGROUND

The history of nuclear medicine over the past 50 years highlights the strong link between investments in chemistry and the development of radionuclides and radiolabeled compounds. In fact, one can trace the major advances in nuclear medicine directly to research in chemistry. These advances have had a major impact on the practice of health care. According to the Society of Nuclear Medicine, 20 million nuclear medicine procedures using radiopharmaceuticals and imaging instruments are carried out in hospitals in the United States alone each year to diagnose disease and to deliver targeted treatments. These techniques have also been adopted by basic and clinical scientists in dozens of fields (e.g., cardiology, oncology, neurology, psychiatry) for diagnosis and as scientific tools. For example, many pharmaceutical companies are now developing radiopharmaceuticals as biomarkers for new drug targets to facilitate the entry of their new drugs into the practice of health care and to objectively examine drug efficacy at a particular target relative to clinical outcome (Erondu et al. 2006). This has created a demand for new radiopharmaceuticals and a corresponding need for chemists and other imaging scientists who are trained to develop them.

6.2 SIGNIFICANT DISCOVERIES

Government investments in chemistry have facilitated the advancement of nuclear medicine, molecular imaging,[1] and targeted radionuclide therapy. For example, research in nuclear chemistry and radiochemistry (Sidebar 6.1), coupled with accelerator technology and engineering, has enabled the introduction of new radionuclides into the practice of medicine. Similarly, progress in synthetic organic and inorganic chemistry laid the groundwork for dozens of compounds labeled with positron emitters or single photon emitters, which are now used in many clinical specialties. These discoveries have resulted from the collaborative efforts of multi-disciplinary teams of scientists and clinician-scientists, ultimately translating new concepts into clinical practice. Three examples are provided in the following sections.

FDG-PET

Tumors and some organs, such as the brain, use glucose as a source of energy. FDG (Sidebar 2.2) is a fluorine-18-labeled derivative of glucose (fluorodeoxyglucose) which is used with positron emission tomography (PET) to provide a map of where glucose is metabolized in the body. Because tumors, as well as the brain and the heart, all use glucose as a source of energy, FDG is widely used in cancer diagnosis and in cardiology, neurology, and

---

[1]Molecular imaging is a scientific discipline that studies new ways of imaging molecular events and biochemical reactions in a living organism using labeled tracers with high molecular specificity.

SIDEBAR 6.1 Disciplines and Specialties within Chemistry

Organic chemistry studies the synthesis, structure and properties of carbon compounds.

Inorganic chemistry studies the chemistry of all elements of the periodic table. Of particular relevance to radiopharmaceutical chemistry is bioinorganic chemistry, which includes coordination chemistry and the incorporation of radio-metals into targeted radiopharmaceuticals.

Radiopharmaceutical chemistry designs, synthesizes, and evaluates chemical compounds that are labeled with a radionuclide. These radiopharmaceutical compounds are used for molecular imaging or for targeted radionuclide therapy (Chapter 4).

Synthetic organic chemistry is one sub-area that is of particular relevance and deals with the design and synthesis of complex molecules. The second is medicinal chemistry, which seeks to design and synthesize new organic compounds to serve as drug candidates, as well as to understand how the compounds interact within living organisms.

Nuclear and radiochemistry studies the chemical properties of radioactive elements to practical applications of radioactivity and nuclear technology.

Combinatorial chemistry is used to generate different combinations of chemicals starting with a subset of compounds. The building blocks may be peptides, nucleic acids or small molecules. The libraries of compounds formed by this methodology are generally used in drug development.

---

psychiatry. FDG is now widely available to hospitals throughout the United States and the world from a network of regional commercial cyclotron/FDG distribution centers (Figure 6.1). With the current large infrastructure of commercial cyclotron/FDG distribution centers, many chemists are developing other highly targeted fluorine-18-labeled compounds to take advantage of this unique network to broaden the use of PET for making health care decisions. The translation of FDG from the chemistry laboratory into a practical clinical tool had its roots in government-supported research in hot atom chemistry (see Chapter 5), cyclotron targetry, biochemistry, synthetic chemistry, nuclear chemistry, and radiochemistry that was integrated with engineering and automation (Fowler and Ido 2002).

Technetium-99m

Technetium-99m is a radionuclide that emits a photon, and this energy is ideally matched to the Anger camera, a device used in nuclear medicine worldwide. Not only is technetium-99m valuable clinically, but it is also practical for routine use, because it is extracted from molybdenum-99,

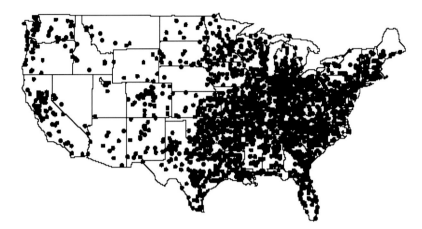

FIGURE 6.1 Map of commercial cyclotron/FDG/radiopharmacies in the United States. SOURCE: Courtesy of Michael Phelps, University of California at Los Angeles.

which has a 66-hour half-life. Greater understanding of the properties of technetium through research spanning over a number of decades (Nicolini and Mazzi 1999) laid the groundwork for developing many technetium-99m labeled radiopharmaceuticals. In parallel to these advances in chemistry, nuclear medicine kits were developed and refined, facilitating the preparation and commercialization of technetium-99m-radiopharmaceuticals (Eckelman and Richards 1970, 1971). These radiopharmaceuticals allow physicians to diagnose life-threatening diseases with great accuracy. The availability of technetium-99m and the radiopharmaceuticals derived from it exemplify the advances in patient care that can result from collaborative efforts among chemists, physicists, and biologists from around the world. Today, technetium-99m is the most widely used radionuclide in nuclear medicine, accounting for more than 70 percent of all procedures (Nuclear Energy Agency 2000).

Targeted Radionuclide Therapy

Targeted radionuclide therapy (see Sidebar 2.3) is a form of treatment that delivers therapeutic doses of radiation to malignant tumors by administering a molecule that is labeled with a radionuclide. For example, alpha particle emitters such as astatine-211 have great appeal for targeted radionuclide therapy because of their high toxicity to the cell and their ability to irradiate tumor volumes in the cellular range (i.e., 50–80 microns). Translation of alpha-particle emitters into the clinical domain has now been accomplished. This could not have occurred without advances in several areas of radiochemistry, including radionuclide production, separations chemistry, and labeling methods that circumvent the problem related to high radiation levels (i.e., radiolysis) generated by therapeutic levels of radionuclide (Zalutsky 2003). Targeted radionuclide therapy is discussed in further detail in Chapter 4.

6.3 CURRENT STATE OF THE FIELD AND EMERGING PRIORITIES

In the pharmaceutical industry and in many clinical specialties—particularly oncology, cardiology, neurology, and psychiatry—there is a demand for new radiopharmaceuticals to advance our knowledge of human biochemistry and physiology and to improve the ability to diagnose and treat diseases. The committee reviewed the current state and trends in radiopharmaceutical research and development (R&D), which are discussed in the following two sections. The first section (6.3.1) summarizes five priority areas with broad public health impact where radiopharmaceuticals could serve as scientific and clinical tools leading to major breakthroughs in health care and basic understanding of human biology. The second section (6.3.2) describes technologies and methods currently being explored that could enable innovations in radiopharmaceutical development and advances in these five priority areas.

6.3.1 Broad Public Health Priorities Enabled by Radiopharmaceutical Technology

1. **Cancer Biology and Targeted Radionuclide Therapy.** Greater understanding of the abnormal biology of tumor cells will allow cancer treatments to be developed that target these features (rather than non-specifically targeting rapidly dividing cells, which is the approach of most chemotherapeutics). Research is needed to develop the following: radiopharmaceuticals that enable an understanding and characterization of abnormal cellular biology to predict the most effective therapy in a particular patient; labeled anti-cancer drugs to determine whether the drug targets the tumor; radiotherapeutic agents to deliver the radionuclide to the tumor; and diagnostic radiopharmaceuticals to monitor response to treatment (Webber 2005).

2. **Neuroscience, Neurology and Psychiatry.** A large fraction of the efforts in radiopharmaceutical chemistry over the past 30 years has been dedicated to understanding the relationship between brain chemistry, behavior, and disease. Although substantial progress has been made in many

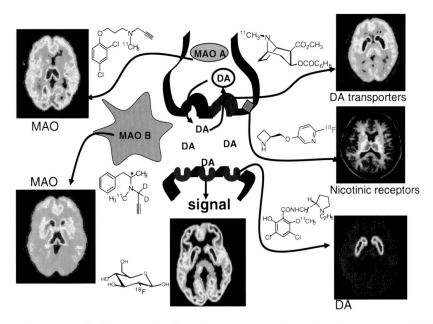

FIGURE 6.2 Radiotracers for imaging neurotransmitter function, as exemplified in the brain dopamine system. A simplified diagram of a dopamine (DA) synapse shows the dopamine transporter (red), dopamine receptors (blue), and monoamine oxidase (MAO) A and B, a nicotine binding site (green), and brain glucose metabolism along with radiotracer structures and human brain images corresponding to each of these molecular targets. SOURCE: Courtesy of Joanna Fowler, Brookhaven National Laboratory.

areas, only a handful of the hundreds of neurotransmitters[2] and metabolic processes that drive brain function can be imaged and quantified with high specificity (Fowler et al. 2003, Kung et al. 2003) (see Figure 6.2). Many more highly targeted radiopharmaceuticals are required to identify the molecular abnormalities of neurodegenerative disorders, such as Alzheimer's and Parkinson's diseases, and psychiatric illnesses, such as schizophrenia and depression, so that better treatments can be developed. In addition, understanding addictive behaviors, such as cigarette smoking and overeating, is essential for the prevention of chronic diseases, such as diabetes, heart disease, and cancer (Bergen and Caporaso 1999, NIMH 2006). These diseases account for much of the morbidity and mortality in the United States and are a major public health burden. The intellectual and techni-

---

[2]Neurotransmitters are chemicals that relay signals between the brain and other cells. Dopamine and serotonin are examples of a neurotransmitter.

cal hurdles of developing the radiotracers of the future are enormous and depend on the stimulation of the flow of new ideas and the development of new technologies (see Section 6.3.2). However, the opportunities that molecular imaging offers to expand our knowledge of the human brain and to integrate this into the development of treatments for mental illness are unprecedented.

3. **Drug Development.** Radiolabeled compounds and imaging technologies are now being used in drug research and development both to measure drug pharmacokinetics and drug pharmacodynamics (Collins and Wahl 2002; also see Chapter 2). This has been stimulated in part by the increasingly prohibitive costs of drug development and the high rate of failure of new drugs entering clinical trials. Radiolabeled compounds can serve as scientific tools for early identification of problems such as poor bioavailability and non-target interactions which can lead to failure later on. In this way molecular imaging offers the potential for accelerating the process of drug discovery while also reducing costs. All large pharmaceutical companies today either have small-animal (microPET) and human PET scanners or relationships with academic and other PET programs that provide these unique scientific tools.

4. **Cardiovascular Disease.** A large fraction of the nuclear medicine tests conducted in the United States is used for cardiology. Single photon emission computed tomography tracers are now widely employed for estimating the severity of heart disease and for defining a patient's future risk of heart attacks and cardiac death. PET tracers have also provided additional gains in accurately diagnosing coronary artery disease, reducing the need for invasive diagnostic procedures, such as coronary angiography. One research priority in cardiology includes identifying techniques for characterizing the functional and biological processes associated with structural alterations in the vessel wall that play a central role in the development of coronary artery disease. Further priorities include developing image-based radionuclide approaches for aiding in the design, implementation, and efficient assessment of gene- and cell-based treatment strategies in cardiovascular disease.

5. **Genetics and Personalized Medicine.** The sequencing of the human genome and new knowledge in proteomics, systems biology,[3] and pathogenesis of human disease offer unprecedented opportunity for the development of new radiopharmaceuticals to image and quantify phenotypic expression of genetic pathology (e.g., upregulated EGF receptors in HER2 mutations). The development of these radiopharmaceuticals will allow scientists to better understand the relationship between genes and normal and abnormal

---

[3]The objective of systems biology is to model the interactions within a biological system and to study how these interactions give rise to the function and behavior of that system.

physiology, and to plan, deliver, and monitor treatment at the level of an individual patient. The identification of new genes and new protein products and their links to specific diseases will continue to generate the need for chemists to create new radiopharmaceuticals.

6.3.2 Specific Technologies and Methods

The demand for new radiopharmaceuticals from many medical specialties particularly oncology, cardiology, neurology, and psychiatry, and especially the pharmaceutical industry, has placed a sense of urgency on stimulating the flow of new ideas and accelerating the pace of development. Currently, chemists working in the areas of molecular imaging and targeted radionuclide therapy are focused on designing and synthesizing radiopharmaceuticals with the required bioavailability and specificity to act as true tracers targeting specific cellular elements (e.g., receptors, enzymes, transporters, antigens, etc.) in healthy human subjects and in patients. Goals are to make labeling chemistry occur faster, more efficiently, and at smaller and smaller scales to give labeled compounds of very high specific activity that can act as true tracers.[4]

Specific activity is a particularly important consideration in the design of molecularly targeted imaging agents and therapeutics. The degree to which improving specific activity must be addressed depends on the nature of the molecular target; specific activity is critical for imaging receptors present at a copy number of 1,000 per cell, but less of an issue with receptors such as the epidermal growth factor receptor that are present at a concentration of millions per cell. Improving specific activity can also be essential for molecules that are exquisitely chemotoxic or can perturb biology at subnanomolar concentrations. We note that the specific activity values described in the literature are generally far below the theoretical values and are highly variable. Thus, identifying and removing sources of carrier in radionuclide production (in cases where the target and the radionuclide are different chemical elements) and in radiotracer synthesis remains one of the major challenges in radiopharmaceutical chemistry.

Two high research priorities that are under investigation are carbon-11 and fluorine-18 chemistry and peptide and antibody labeling. Research in these areas has been stimulated by the increased utilization of PET and the promise of targeted radionuclide therapy. Fluorine-18 radiopharmaceuticals and antibody and peptide radiopharmaceuticals each have their own specific sets of challenges and needs which are further described in Sidebars 6.2 and 6.3. In addition, radiopharmaceuticals labeled with gallium-68 (a

---

[4]A tracer is a measurable substance used to mimic, follow, or trace a chemical compound or element without perturbing the process.

**SIDEBAR 6.2 Fluorine-18 Radiopharmaceutical
Chemistry Needs**

Fluorine-18 [F-18]-labeled compounds are expected to play a large role in the future of nuclear medicine because of the relatively long half-life of F-18 and the large network of cyclotron/radiopharmacy distribution centers operating throughout the United States from which they can be obtained (see Figure 6.1). To advance the development and translation of F-18-labeled compounds, the following are needed:

- Efficient methods to concentrate F-18 from cyclotron targets;
- Improved specific activity of F-18 fluoride and F-18 compounds;
- High-yield reactions to give F-18 aryl fluorides for activated and non-activated rings;
- More reactive synthetic precursors for F-18 labeling;
- Improvements in stability of carbon-halogen bonds;
- Efficient chemistry (including high-yield labeling of an F-18 synthon) to label peptides, antibodies and other large molecules; and
- Development of a reliable, one-step nucleophilic synthesis of F-18-DOPA from F-18 fluoride.

---

positron emitter that is available from the Ge-68/Ga-68 generator) are used for receptor imaging and research purposes in a large number of clinical diagnostic and therapeutic applications throughout Europe (Antunes et al. 2007). Although experience with Ga-68 labeled tracers in the United States is limited, this radionuclide and the radiopharmaceuticals labeled with it deserve attention, because the generator for Ga-68 is convenient to use and the resulting radiopharmaceuticals could be distributed to the large network of facilities with stand-alone PET cameras for clinical imaging.

In addition to performing research directed toward radiotracer synthesis, chemists also design radiotracers and investigate the mechanisms underlying the distribution and kinetics of labeled compounds in living systems. This type of work addresses a major obstacle in radiotracer R&D—namely, the lack of knowledge for predicting which radiolabeled compounds will have the bioavailability, specificity, and kinetics required to image and quantify specific molecular targets in vivo or to target tumor tissue while sparing healthy organs. In this regard, progress in understanding and reducing non-specific binding would be a major advance. Of particular importance is research on the design and development of radiotracers that are more broadly applicable to common pathophysiological processes, which may be more useful and more readily commercialized (e.g., targets involved

---

**SIDEBAR 6.3 Antibody/Peptide
Radiopharmaceutical Chemistry Needs**

A central issue in the advancement of targeted radionuclide therapy lies in the design and development of labeled antibodies and peptides that target the tumor and spare healthy tissues. Chemistry plays a major role in this process, and the research priorities identified by the committee with input from experts are as follows:

• To better understand how the chelating agent,[a] radionuclide, and conjugation method contribute to behavior in vivo;
• To design radiolabeled ligands with better in vivo properties (faster blood clearance, cleavable linkers for renal clearance);
• To retain the desired targeting properties of the parent compound after labeling;
• To develop smaller, less polar,[b] kinetically stable radiometal ligand complexes that are readily available;
• To develop processing and purification methods to reliably produce high-specific-activity radionuclides;
• To synthesize more probes with higher affinity for targeting and capture, and smaller capture agents bearing the radionuclide that attach to the carrier for pre-targeting;
• To advance radiopharmaceutical applications of the germanium-68/gallium-68 generator to take advantage of the availability of this generator and PET; and
• To develop methods to produce clinical and commercial quantities of therapeutic radionuclides and to increase the availability of radionuclides approved by the Food and Drug Administration.

---

[a]Chelation is a chemical process whereby a chelating agent binds to a metal ion, forming a metal complex known as a chelate.
[b]A chemical compound is made up of one or more chemical bonds between atoms. How the bonds share electrons between the bonds will determine a compound's polarity. In a polar compound, such as water, there is unequal sharing of the electrons creating a slightly positively charged end and a slightly negatively charged end.

---

in inflammation and infection, angiogenesis, tissue hypoxia, mitochondrial targets, cell signaling targets, and targets associated with diabetes, obesity, metabolic syndrome, or liver disease).

To meet these intellectual and technical challenges, a new molecular imaging radiotracer discovery and development process needs to be developed based on modern genomics, proteomics, and systems biology and driven by the invention of new molecular technology platforms to synthesize, label, and biologically screen in vitro for translation from a good scientific base to animal models and patients. This process should focus on being a measurement science, not on clinical diagnostics, even though that is the end objective through the measurements that result. Molecular diagnostics and molecular therapeutics are desperately in need of biochemical, biological, and pharmacological measurements of disease in vivo and in patients to guide the discovery and development of new generations of more effective and personalized drugs. To keep pace with these clinical and research demands, nuclear medicine researchers are also seeing innovation in automation. For example, technologies that will provide simple, inexpensive modules for making carbon-11 labeled precursors and for automating other routine operations (e.g., quality control) are being developed. Furthermore, as noted in Chapter 2, microfluidic and microchip technologies are expected to advance this field (Figure 6.3)[5] (Lee et al. 2005). Emerging areas such as nanosciences,[6] advanced materials sciences,[7] and strategically designed combinatorial libraries[8] will also play an integral role in driving both radiopharmaceutical design and automation.

Although there is a need to develop new radiopharmaceuticals for new molecular targets, it is important to note that there are many highly promising radionuclides, precursor molecules, and radiopharmaceuticals that are not readily available to institutions without an infrastructure for isotope production or radiopharmaceutical chemistry. These include fluorine-18-fluoro-L-dihydroxyphenylalanine (FDOPA), fluorine-18-fluoro-L-thymidine (FLT), copper-64-diacetyl-bis(N4-methyl-thiosemicarbazone (ATSM), iodine-123-meta-iodobenzylguanidine (MIBG), fluorine-18-fluorocholine, fluorine-18-fallypride, fluorine-18-fluoroprophyl-β–carbomethyoxy-3β-(4-iodophenyltropane) (FP-CIT), Quadramet®, Therasphere®, copper-64-DOTA peptides, copper-62-generator, fluorine-18-fluoride, iodine-124 labeled antibodies, peptides, and targeted therapy drugs that inhibit signal transduction molecules. Thus, there is a need to increase the availability of specialized radiopharmaceuticals both for clinical diagnosis and treatment and also as research tools in the exploration of novel applications (in the "bench-to-bedside-and-back trajectory"). For example, MIBG, used

---

[5]Microfluidics is a multi-disciplinary field that studies how fluids behave at microliter and nanoliter volume and the design of systems in which small volumes of fluids will be used to provide automated sample processing, synthesis, separation, and measurements in devices commonly termed lab-on-a chip (see Chapter 2). For example, it is used in procedures such as in DNA analysis.

[6]Nanoscience is the study of atoms, molecules, and objects whose size is between 1 and 100 nanometers.

[7]Materials science is an inter-disciplinary field comprising applied physics, chemistry, and engineering that studies the physical properties of matter and its applications.

[8]Combinatorial libraries are sets of compounds prepared using combinatorial chemistry (see Sidebar 6.1). These libraries allow scientists to access a wide range of substances and to search for compounds that bind to specific biological and non-biological targets. For example, when a molecule is added to the library, some of the compounds in the library will bind to it, enabling the discovery of individual compounds that recognize that molecule.

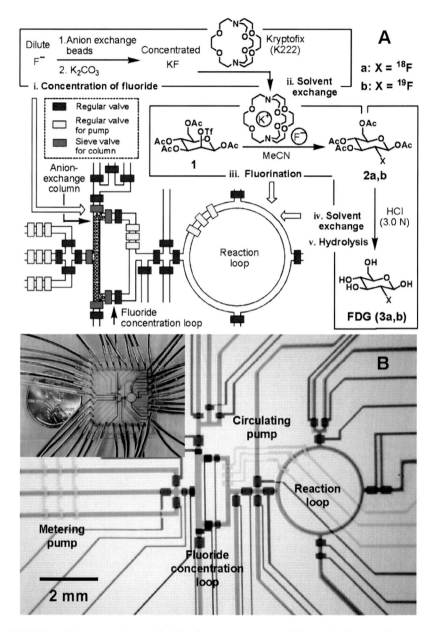

FIGURE 6.3 Integrated microfluidics for the synthesis of FDG. (A) Schematic representation of a chemical reaction circuit used in the production of FDG. (B) Optical micrograph of the central area of the circuit. SOURCE: Lee et al. 2005. Reprinted with permission from the American Association for the Advancement of Science.

initially mainly for assessment of neuroendocrine tumors, is now showing promise in early diagnosis of heart failure, a major health and economic issue in the United States. It is important to keep in mind that any new developments in targeted radionuclide therapy require access to research radionuclides (see Chapters 4 and 5).

6.4 CURRENT NEEDS AND IMPEDIMENTS

Although the scientific opportunities and medical challenges have never been more exciting and the demand for new radiopharmaceuticals has never been greater, the nuclear medicine infrastructure on which future innovation and discovery depend hangs in the balance. Four major impediments—some of which are elaborated further in other chapters of the report—stand in the way of scientific and medical progress and the competitive edge that the United States has held for more than 50 years:

1. **Lack of Support for Radiopharmaceutical R&D.** The committee finds that as a result of the reduction in funding from the U.S. Department of Energy-Office of Biological and Environmental Research (DOE-OBER) has seen a substantial loss of support for basic radiopharmaceutical chemistry research. This includes methodological research in synthetic chemistry, yield optimization, purification strategies, structure-activity relationships, radionuclide and targetry research, and preclinical and clinical evaluation. In addition, there is no support for infrastructures (accelerators, imaging instruments) that are the underpinning of radiopharmaceutical development.

2. **Shortage of Trained Chemists and Physician Scientists** (see Chapter 8). One of the most enriching aspects of radiopharmaceutical research is that it is generally carried out in an interdisciplinary environment where chemists, physicists, engineers, biologists, and physicians work together sharing the excitement of solving important problems in medicine. However, there is a critical shortage of trained chemists (typically, synthetic chemists with expertise in nuclear chemistry and radiochemistry are needed) for radiotracer and radiopharmaceutical R&D. This is a major impediment that has been documented in multiple reports over the past 20 years (e.g., DOE 2002, NRC 2007). There is also a lack of trained physician-scientists who are able to provide the expertise to collaborate in the basic clinical feasibility studies required to translate promising radiopharmaceuticals to the clinic.

3. **Inappropriate Regulatory Requirements** (see Chapter 4). Because the ultimate goal in radiopharmaceutical R&D is to use radiopharmaceuticals as scientific and clinical tools to investigate the systems biology of disease in healthy human subjects and patients, obtaining approval to

evaluate promising new labeled compounds in humans is essential. Currently, this is a bottleneck, stifling innovation and driving many research groups to carry out their initial evaluations of new radiopharmaceuticals with collaborators in other countries. A regulatory framework specific for radiopharmaceuticals that will facilitate the rapid and safe translation of radiopharmaceuticals from animals to humans for clinical feasibility studies is clearly needed.

4. **Limited Radionuclide Availability** (see Chapter 5). There is no dedicated domestic high energy accelerator for R&D and training for the development of the radionuclides of the future and for year-round production of medical radionuclides. These are needed not only for developing and evaluating the targeted radiotherapeutic agents, but also for production of some largely unexplored PET tracers. Radionuclides that are available intermittently from DOE labs are expensive due to full cost recovery requirements preventing their development for nuclear medicine.

6.5 RECOMMENDATIONS

The committee formulated two recommendations to meet the future needs for radiopharmaceutical development for the diagnosis and treatment of human disease and to overcome national impediments to their entry into the practice of health care.

RECOMMENDATION 1: Enhance the federal commitment to nuclear medicine research. Given the somewhat different orientations of the DOE and the National Institutes of Health (NIH) toward nuclear medicine research, the two agencies should find some cooperative mechanism to support radionuclide production and distribution; basic research in radionuclide production, nuclear imaging, radiopharmaceutical/radiotracer and therapy development; and the transfer of these technologies into routine clinical use.

> **Implementation Action 1A1:** A national nuclear medicine research program should be coordinated by the DOE and NIH, with the former emphasizing the general development of technology and the latter disease-specific applications.

> **Implementation Action 1A2:** In developing their strategic plan, the agencies should avail themselves of advice from a broad range of authorities in academia, national laboratories and industry; these authorities should include experts in physics, engineering, chemistry, radiopharmaceutical science, commercial development, regulatory affairs, clinical trials, and radiation biology.

RECOMMENDATION 2: *Encourage interdisciplinary collaboration. DOE-OBER should support collaborations between basic chemistry and physics laboratories, as well as multi-disciplinary centers focused on nuclear medicine technology development and application, to stimulate the flow of new ideas for the development of next-generation radiopharmaceuticals and imaging instrumentation.*

7

Instrumentation and Computational Sciences

This chapter addresses the second charge to the committee to provide findings and recommendations regarding "future needs for computational and instrument development for more precise localization of radiotracers in normal and aberrant cell physiologies." The content of this chapter, particularly of the sections delineating future needs, includes information and opinions derived from discussions with physicists, engineers, and mathematicians working in both industry and academia.

The chapter is divided into the following six sections:

- Background (7.1),
- Significant Discoveries (7.2),
- Current State of the Field and Emerging Priorities (7.3),
- Future Needs (7.4),
- Findings (7.5), and
- Recommendations (7.6).

7.1 BACKGROUND

As discussed in other chapters of this report, the use of nuclear medicine technology for both diagnostic and therapeutic applications is central to the goal of personalized medicine. A key component of nuclear medicine is the quantitative imaging of radiopharmaceutical distributions. Imaging scientists often classify imaging tasks into two main categories: the detection task and the estimation task. The goal of detection is to see if some-

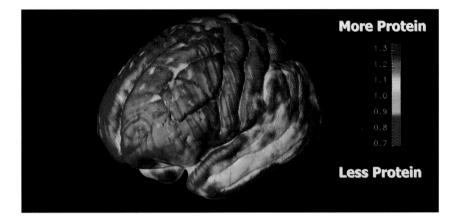

FIGURE 7.1 Parametric image of brain that shows the progression of abnormality of proteins in patients with Alzheimer's disease. SOURCE: Courtesy of Henry Huang, UCLA.

thing is present (i.e., reading an image and making a diagnosis based on where the activity is located and the relative accumulation of the radiotracer to other tissues), and the goal of the estimation task is to determine how much of it is present (e.g., to measure the rate of glucose metabolism from a fluorine-18 fluorodeoxyglucose (FDG)-positron emission tomography (PET) study). The first step to achieve these goals is to acquire the data by accurately measuring the activity of the radioactive tracer in the patient. Once the data are acquired, image reconstruction algorithms are required to generate tomographic image sets of the spatial distribution of radiotracer within the body.

Recent developments involve modeling the physical characteristics of the camera into the iterative reconstruction process to improve image quality and radionuclide quantification. Finally, in addition to basic image display and analysis tools, advanced compartmental modeling tools are needed for those applications in which it is necessary to relate tracer uptake kinetics to physiologic or biochemical measures such as perfusion or receptor concentration, etc. (see Figure 7.1). Thus nuclear medicine imaging will gain from a continuum of improvements. These range from advances in solid-state materials for radiation detectors to increase sensitivity,[1] faster

---

[1]Sensitivity of the instrument is defined as the percentage of radioactive decays that are detected. The sensitivity of a scanner depends on a number of factors, including geometric solid angle coverage and efficiency of the detectors. For single photon emission computed tomography (SPECT) the sensitivity also depends on the collimator, which is needed to define the direction of the gamma ray.

scintillators for higher count rate performance and time-of-flight (TOF) applications, and higher light output for improved aperture, and maximum image quality and tracer quantification with the integration of tracer kinetic models into the workstation toolkit.

To meet these goals, the development of imaging instruments and computational tools requires collaborative teams of investigators in physics, engineering, and mathematics who understand the entire process of nuclear medicine image generation. This ranges from understanding radionuclide decay (from simple single photon and positron emitters such as technetium-99m and fluorine-18 to complex isotope decays such as iodine-124 with positrons and prompt gamma emissions, which complicate signal acquisition in the 511-keV window), to the attenuation and scatter properties in the patient, to single photon and PET detector characteristics, to gamma camera and PET scanner performance, image reconstruction, processing, and finally image registration and display tools.

Starting with basic detector technologies, there has been (and continues to be) a natural synergy between the nuclear medicine detector/scanner development teams and basic nuclear and high-energy physics groups. As is discussed in Section 7.2, many of the nuclear medicine instruments used in the clinic today had their roots in the nuclear and high-energy physics laboratories that were developing advanced detectors to investigate the nucleus and structure of matter. For example, the most important annual meeting for the science and engineering of nuclear medicine instrumentation and imaging techniques is the Institute of Electrical and Electronics Engineers (IEEE) Nuclear Science Symposium and Medical Imaging Conference, which is a joint conference between nuclear medicine physics and instrumentation development teams and high-energy physics groups. It is at this meeting that the leading-edge technologies in radiation detectors are presented, frequently providing the impetus for innovations in nuclear medicine equipment. Those in attendance include physicists, engineers, and scientists from universities, national laboratories, and industry, and the atmosphere is one of multidisciplinary collaboration to bring new technologies into improved clinical instrumentation.

SPECT and PET cameras are highly integrated pieces of equipment that rely on the optimization of multiple subsystems to achieve peak performance. In SPECT, this requires high-quality crystal manufacture, collimator design, high-quantum-efficiency photomultiplier tubes, fast signal processing electronics, integrated gating for cardiac applications, advanced image processing tools, and so on. Weakness in any one of these components substantially affects the final image quality. As the field moves to earlier detection of cancer and neurological and cardiac diseases, pressure is exerted on scientists and equipment manufacturers to improve the limits of detectability of nuclear imaging devices (through improvements in both resolution and sensitivity), and to incorporate new technology that will achieve this objective in the clinical imaging equipment of today, so that it is reliable, practical, and easy to use.

7.2 SIGNIFICANT DISCOVERIES

Federal investments in instrumentation and computational development have included infrastructure support at the national laboratories as well as direct grants to universities and national laboratories from the Department of Energy (DOE), the National Science Foundation, and the National Institutes of Health (NIH). Almost all of the core technologies in instrumentation and computation used in nuclear medicine have been developed as a result of the Atomic Energy Commission (AEC) and the DOE funding (see Chapter 2). Some of the key developments include the Anger camera (the basic foundation for all single photon imaging systems currently in use), SPECT, PET, cyclotron targetry and radionuclide generator systems, basic image reconstruction algorithms, and kinetic modeling applied to PET and SPECT studies.

The state-of-the-art SPECT and PET scanners used today in the clinic illustrate how critical it is to have the infrastructure and funding to support the flow of technology from the nuclear and high-energy laboratories that develop new detectors and electronics to the nuclear medicine instrumentation laboratories that develop new imaging tools. Often these basic science experiments are large efforts that utilize the expertise of many individuals at the national laboratories with contributions from university-based basic research groups. There are many examples of projects that were promising but high risk, and development of these projects was undertaken by DOE-funded laboratories which had the time and expertise to work on the new technologies over many years. DOE's mission to develop new technologies for imaging allowed for long-range (i.e., more than 5-year), high-risk projects with an emphasis on basic instrumentation research. In contrast, NIH's mission is to carry out more short-term (2 to 5 years), lower-risk (i.e., more preliminary data) projects that emphasize the integration or evaluation of new technologies for clinical application. The long-range view of DOE support allowed time for the investigator to pursue alternative approaches, some of which failed, in search of the most practical solution.

To illustrate this flow of technology, we note two of the many examples of technology development in PET instrumentation that were funded by DOE, as neither was a good candidate for NIH funding, and that were later commercialized. The first is the University of Pennsylvania's PennPET scanner project. The PennPET project developed scanners designed for clinical use that were based on Anger-logic detectors (similar in concept to the Anger camera developed earlier at UC Radiation Laboratory with AEC funding) and fully three-dimensional data acquisition and image reconstruction. This technology was commercialized by UGM Medical Systems in the early 1990s, and later marketed by General Electric, ADAC Laboratories, and Philips Medical Systems.

The second example is the University of California at Los Angeles (UCLA) microPET scanner project. The UCLA microPET scanner was the first PET scanner to utilize lutetium oxyorthosilicate (LSO), a material that has since become the scintillator of choice for many clinical scanners. Moreover, it set a precedent for dedicated, high-resolution, small animal imaging scanners (see Figure 7.2) that was commercialized by Concorde Microsystems in the late 1990s. This has helped initiate the recent growth of preclinical research with imaging of small animals (e.g., mice and rats) to study disease and develop new pharmaceuticals for monitoring and treatment (see Figure 7.3). Today there are at least 200 scanners installed by a variety of vendors, half of which can be found in pharmaceutical industrial laboratories.

While DOE funding is responsible for many of the basic technologies used in PET and SPECT instrumentation today, NIH has also played a critical role. The funding expended by NIH for research has demonstrated the clinical utility and application of these technologies. A prime example is the recent development of PET/computed tomography (CT) scanners. Although the principles are based on PET technologies developed at DOE-funded laboratories, the first prototype PET/CT scanner was developed in the late 1990s as a result of an NIH grant at the University of Pittsburgh in collaboration with CTI PET Systems. That work demonstrated the immediate

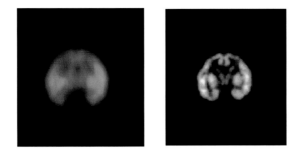

FIGURE 7.2 Comparison of images of a baby rhesus monkey brain phantom obtained with a clinical scanner (left) and a microPET scanner (right) illustrates the improvement in spatial resolution possible with a dedicated small animal scanner. SOURCE: Courtesy of Arion Chatziioannou, UCLA Crump Institute for Molecular Imaging.

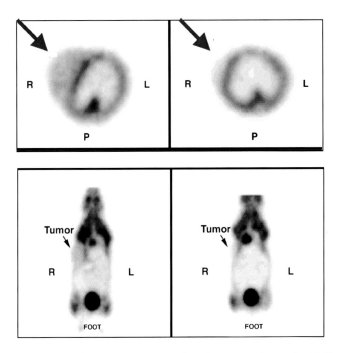

FIGURE 7.3 Images of a mammary tumor-bearing mouse imaged with fluorine-18-FDG following oncogene induction. The mouse was imaged first while doxycycline was being administered (left) and then 2 days later after doxycycline was turned off (right). Note decreased activity in tumor (at arrow) in second study. SOURCE: Courtesy of Lewis Chodosh, University of Pennsylvania.

impact of PET/CT in clinical oncology and the commercial sector rapidly developed these imaging instruments for clinical practice. In fact, all PET scanners today are marketed as PET/CT scanners because the combination of anatomic information (CT) and physiological information (PET) has proved to be essential for clinical diagnosis.

A similar story holds true for single photon emission computed tomography (SPECT)/CT scanners. The basic technical principles of SPECT were developed as a result of DOE funding at the University of Pennsylvania and Duke University. However, it was funding from NIH in the 1990s to the University of California at San Francisco that supported the research that integrated SPECT with CT (see Figure 7.4).

TOF PET is another example of a technology that is now available commercially as a result of funding from DOE through the 1980s and 1990s, and, more recently, funding from the National Institute of Bio-

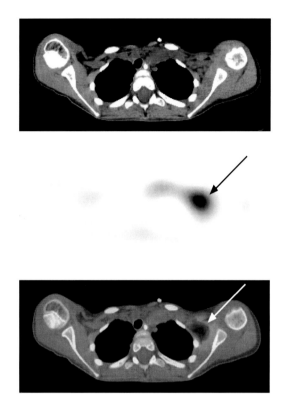

FIGURE 7.4 Neuroblastoma imaged with 131-I-meta-iodobenzylguanidine (MIBG) on a combined SPECT/CT instrument illustrates the benefit of correlating the functional data with the anatomical data. Top image is CT, middle image is SPECT, bottom image is combined SPECT/CT showing SPECT and CT in different colors. SOURCE: Reprinted by permission of the Society of Nuclear Medicine from Tang et al. 2001.

medical Imaging and Bioengineering. Its development took over 25 years to transition from the laboratory to the clinic since it required the combination of new developments of scintillators, electronics, and image reconstruction, which illustrates the need for long-term funding and involvement of different funding agencies. In 2006, TOF finally was introduced in a commercial product by Philips Medical Systems. Its advantage in cancer detection and staging has been demonstrated in terms of superior image quality (higher contrast with lower noise for the same number of events detected) and better detection of lesions compared to conventional PET (see Figure 7.5), particularly in heavy patients.

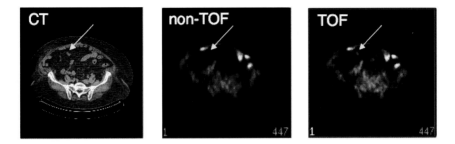

FIGURE 7.5 Colon cancer patient (119 kg) imaged with fluorine-18-FDG illustrating improvement in lesion detectability with TOF compared to conventional (non-TOF) PET for the same number of detected events and the same number of iterations in the reconstruction algorithm. The data were reconstructed without TOF information (middle) and with TOF information (right) and compared to low-dose CT image (left) acquired immediately beforehand on combined PET/CT instrument. Note the TOF reconstruction shows higher uptake and better definition of the lesion (at arrow). SOURCE: Courtesy of Joel Karp, University of Pennsylvania.

7.3 CURRENT STATE OF THE FIELD AND EMERGING PRIORITIES

Emerging goals for nuclear medicine include early detection, which will require improvements in equipment sensitivity; the accurate quantification of biomarker uptake in disease for the evaluation of treatment response; and the quantification of radiotracer heterogeneity, which may be of potential utility for dose-painting applications of intensity-modulated radiotherapy. These limits may be tested in preclinical equipment such as microSPECT and microPET scanners, which operate at the cutting edge of the technology, with volumetric resolutions that are approximately 10-fold higher than their counterpart systems in the clinic. For example, the spatial resolution requirements to conduct meaningful preclinical research in mice are much more stringent than those required to conduct clinical studies in patients. To illustrate, a simple argument can be made that since the mouse brain volume is about 1/1,700th the volume of the human brain, we should scale the linear spatial resolution of a human scanner by a factor of 12 in each of the three dimensions to achieve a comparable resolution for mouse brain imaging. With current state-of-the-art technology for human brain imaging, 2.4-mm linear spatial resolution can be achieved with a dedicated brain scanner. To be able to achieve a similar linear spatial resolution in mice, the target is to reach a linear spatial resolution of 0.2 mm. To date, the best linear spatial resolution achieved for small-animal imaging in PET with a commercial instrument is 1.2 mm, which is still a factor of 6 too high (i.e., a factor of 216 in terms of volumetric resolution). Some university-based developmental systems have achieved resolutions of 0.7 mm, but the goal of reaching less than 0.5 mm will require considerable technological development both in detector technology and image reconstruction algorithms. Such improvements in the spatial resolution of microPET systems are not impossible, and are governed by the minification of detector elements, light collection, and image processing software. In addition, methods to overcome depth-of-interaction (DOI) effects, which reduce spatial resolution of small bore scanners for points off central axis, are under development using phoswich and other detector technologies.

The sensitivity of state-of-the-art animal PET scanners is currently 5 percent (Myers and Hume 2002). However, to measure kinetics of tracers with low specific activity requires the development of new techniques than can increase sensitivity to 10 to 20 percent. Detector designs utilizing nonradioactive crystalline materials are advantageous because the high background signal associated with the current LSO crystals places limits on the detection of micrometastatic disease. Furthermore, improved algorithms that can stably reconstruct the activity distribution from low-count statistics will be important.

One advantage of PET compared to SPECT is that the spatial resolution and sensitivity are decoupled. It is very challenging to improve spatial resolution in SPECT without reducing sensitivity because of the basic need for collimation. Although superior spatial resolution has been achieved in SPECT for small-animal imaging using pinhole collimation (<0.5 mm), this has been reached at the cost of sensitivity and field-of-view. Although this trade-off is well suited for brain imaging of a mouse, current technology does not enable this level of performance for body imaging, or for larger animals.

Although great advances have been made in basic nuclear medicine imaging in both the detection and estimation tasks, personalized medicine (Sidebar 2.5) is a challenging goal. It requires the ability to detect many different signals that are specific to a patient's disease. That requirement has led to the increasing development of hybrid imaging systems. Combining a high-spatial-resolution anatomical modality, such as CT, with a high sensitivity molecular imaging modality, such as PET or SPECT, has had a major impact on the current practice of medicine. For example, PET/CT scanners have been rapidly adopted in oncology in diagnosis and treatment planning. Some laboratories and equipment vendors have active research programs to develop PET/MRI scanners (see Figure 7.6).

Another new and exciting technology under development is the Silicon Photomultiplier (SiPM) device. SiPM devices have the potential to offer a low-cost, high-performance photon sensor for use in a wide variety of gamma-ray imaging systems. These devices were originally developed for high-energy physics experiments but are now being tested in both physics

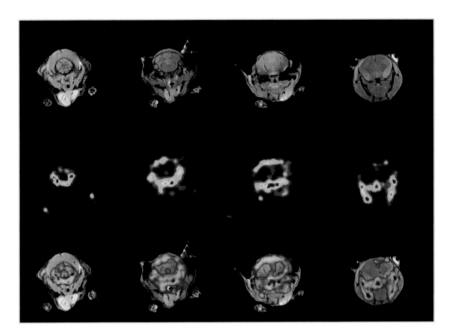

FIGURE 7.6 Simultaneous PET/MR images of mouse brain. The MR image (top row) shows both bone and tissue in the head of the mouse, whereas the PET image (middle row) for this particular study highlights mainly the bony structures of the jaw and skull of the mouse since the data were acquired using fluorine-18-fluoride. An overlay of images and correlation of both modalities is shown in the bottom row, with PET and MR in different colors. SOURCE: Reprinted by permission of the Society of Nuclear Medicine from Cantana et al. 2006.

and nuclear medicine imaging research laboratories for future imaging instruments. Although the potential is already apparent, the use of these devices in imaging instruments has many challenges and risks, and long-term research funding will be required to bring this technology to the clinic. This is also an example of a technology that requires early collaboration between academia and industry during the development phase, since the eventual solution for medical imaging detectors will require input into the design of the photon sensor. Development of SiPMs is ongoing at both large companies (e.g., Hamamatsu) and small companies (e.g., Zecotek, SensL, and Photonique), but it is currently difficult to fund this type of research at universities or national laboratories.

Hand-in-hand with the development of detectors, electronics, and imaging instruments goes the development of image reconstruction algorithms, simulation tools, and techniques for kinetic model analysis. Development of these software tools is essential to accurately model the data and thereby quantify the radiotracer uptake in nuclear medicine studies. The ability to perform this task in practice has benefited from the increased availability of powerful computing resources. For example, an iterative image reconstruction algorithm with data corrections built into the system model was considered to be impractical a decade ago. Yet, this type of algorithm can now be used to generate images in a practical amount of time in both the research laboratory and the clinic (Figures 7.7 and 7.8).

7.4 FUTURE NEEDS

Leaders in instrumentation and computational development in nuclear medicine from universities, national laboratories, and industry were solicited for commentary and analysis. Based on discussions with these experts

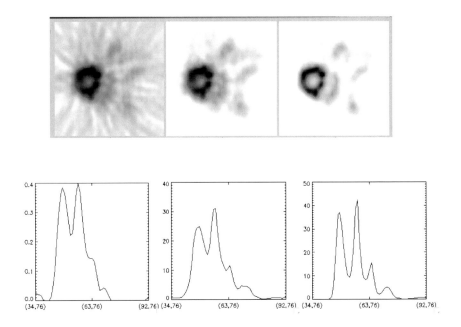

FIGURE 7.7 Images of mouse heart illustrate improvements due to image reconstruction: (left) filtered backprojection algorithm, (middle) iterative ordered-set expectation maximization (OSEM) algorithm, (right) OSEM with detector response modeling. Note that the OSEM reconstruction with detector response modeling has the lowest noise and the best definition of myocardial uptake. SOURCE: Courtesy of Thomas Lewellen, University of Washington.

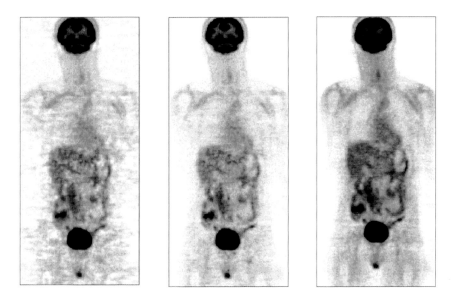

FIGURE 7.8 Images of clinical patient illustrate improvements due to image reconstruction: (left) filtered backprojection algorithm, (middle) iterative OSEM algorithm, (right) OSEM with detector response modeling. Note that the OSEM reconstruction with detector response modeling has the lowest noise and overall best image quality. SOURCE: Courtesy of Paul Kinahan, University of Washington.

as well as committee members' own experiences, the committee concluded that improvements in instrumentation and computation are necessary to lead to advances in quantitative imaging and, in turn, nuclear medicine. These improvements depend on the following:

- better spatial resolution;
- higher sensitivity;
- further integration of instruments to provide multimodality (multisignal) imaging;
- increased coupling of detector and electronics design with image reconstruction; and
- development of clinically robust software tools for data processing and analysis.

The opportunities afforded by improvements in instrumentation and computation could include the following:

- The development of new technology platforms (e.g., integrated microfluidics chips and other automated chemistry and biological screening technologies and nanotechnologies) that would accelerate, diversify, and lower the cost of discovering and validating new molecular imaging probes, biomarkers, surrogate markers, and labeled drugs, as well as new radiotherapeutic agents.

- The invention of new miniaturized particle-accelerator and associated technologies to develop small, low-cost electronic generators for producing short-lived radioisotopes for local use in research and clinical programs. DOE has the largest accelerator technology program in the world, including novel miniaturized accelerator technologies in the DOE weapons program.

- The invention of new detector technologies for PET and SPECT that would enhance sensitivity as well as spatial and temporal resolution. All the successful detectors in PET and SPECT today came from the physics programs of DOE. New base detector materials and detection logic are needed to invent new generations of PET and SPECT imaging systems.

- The development of new iterative algorithms and high-speed/high-capacity computational systems for rapid image reconstruction; this would allow image data to be converted to quantitative parametric images pertaining to biological and pharmacological processes in disease.

7.5 FINDINGS

1. Synergistic collaborations between national laboratories and universities have led to the successful transition of technology from the basic physics laboratory to both biological research and clinical settings. Furthermore, the collaborations between the DOE-funded laboratories and the NIH-funded laboratories have illustrated the value of funding from different agencies with different missions. However, with the loss of nuclear medicine funding from the DOE Office of Biological and Environmental Research (DOE-OBER) in FY 2006, the amount being spent on basic instrument development has fallen from $6.3 million to only $1.9 million (DOE 2006), limiting the ability to explore new and innovative technology solutions.

2. Developments in nuclear imaging instrumentation directly provide tangible benefits for the emerging field of molecular imaging. Three examples of these upcoming technologies include TOF PET, combined PET/MR machines, and SPECT/CT with the potential to allow quantification of single photon radiotracers for the first time; these three technologies will directly impact future patient management in the following ways:

- TOF PET allows significant improvements in clinical image

quality, in particular for large patients (>250 pounds), where current three-dimensional PET scanners are frequently of borderline quality. Further advances in timing resolution beyond the current 600 picoseconds of the Philips Gemini TOF will be coupled to further improvements in signal-to-noise ratio, image contrast, and reduced partial volume corrections, allowing more accurate tracer quantification in small structures.

• Advances in the technology of hybrid scanners will combine the benefits of the soft tissue anatomy, MR spectroscopy, and functional MR alongside the sensitivity of PET imaging. This has the potential to revolutionize imaging of the brain, and with it spur interest in body PET/MR systems for imaging the prostate where spectroscopy is well developed.

• Advances in SPECT/CT instruments will directly facilitate quantitative SPECT studies, of vital importance in targeted radionuclide therapies. Software is under development to co-register serial SPECT/CT exams and generate dosimetric maps for the radionuclide, of significant importance for patient-specific targeted therapy planning. The extensive portfolio of SPECT agents approved by the Food and Drug Administration coupled with the unique ability of SPECT to perform simultaneous multienergy window exams widens previously untapped opportunities in single photon nuclear medicine imaging, through advances in quantitative SPECT imaging.

The above examples represent only a portion of the advances that are likely to be seen in molecular imaging instrumentation over the next decade.

7.6 RECOMMENDATIONS

RECOMMENDATION: *Encourage interdisciplinary collaboration. The DOE-OBER should continue to encourage collaborations between basic chemistry, physics, computer science, and imaging laboratories, as well as multi-disciplinary centers focused on nuclear medicine technology development and application, to stimulate the flow of new ideas for the development and translation of next-generation radiopharmaceuticals and imaging instrumentation. The role of industry should be considered and mechanisms developed that would hasten the technology development process.*

8

Education and Training of Nuclear Medicine Personnel

This chapter addresses part of the fourth charge of the statement of task that requests that the committee examine the "impact of shortages of highly trained radiopharmaceutical chemists and other nuclear medicine scientists on nuclear medicine basic and translational research, drug discovery, patient care, and short- and long-term strategies to alleviate these shortages if they exist."

The chapter is organized into the following sections:

- Background (8.1),
- Current State of the Workforce (8.2),
- Findings (8.3), and
- Recommendations (8.4).

8.1 BACKGROUND

The renaissance of nuclear medicine brought about by the promise of using molecular targets as more precise determinants of disease has created new and greater demands for those providing the basic science expertise for the discipline. Creation of new agents will require interdisciplinary teams of molecular, cellular, and structural biologists, bioinformatics specialists, and synthetic and radiopharmaceutical chemists. Improved instrumentation of combined-modality imaging for humans and animals will rely on highly specialized medical physicists and engineers. The maintenance of contemporary, cyclotron-based research and clinical facilities will require additional radiochemists, radiopharmacists, and physicists, whether located in academic medical centers, government laboratories, or pharmaceutical and biotechnology companies. Add to this list the need for appropriate research training for clinician-scientists, and the future demands for education and training will be extensive.

Moreover, the current exacting needs of research, and to some extent of clinical practice, require a degree of super-specialization on the part of the nuclear medicine community previously unrealized. As examples of this specialization, determining how to target specific receptors in the brain, understanding how mutated forms of protein kinases[1] are involved in cancer, and understanding how to use gene replacement to repair the ailing heart will necessitate a deeper understanding of the biology of disease and its molecular manifestations than ever before. Thus, there are qualitative questions about training candidates for careers in nuclear medicine research as well as quantitative ones that relate to the need for additional specialists.

Because of the multidisciplinary nature of nuclear medicine research and clinical practice, the committee undertook a broad look at the required personnel, from research technologists to clinician-scientists. The committee conducted an extensive search for specific data (e.g., number of faculty positions available, number of positions available in industry, the time it takes to fill each position); however, the committee was unable to find any systematic survey that gave reliable data. To gain a better understanding of the challenges, the committee solicited input from relevant scientific societies, government agencies, and industry representatives. In addition to the comments from scientific societies and government agencies and industry, selected members of training programs for chemists, radiopharmacists, medical physicists, health physicists, and clinician-scientists were invited to a panel discussion at the committee's third meeting (Appendix A) which was dedicated to training needs. The following sections discuss the current status of the workforce by occupation.

8.2 CURRENT STATUS OF THE WORKFORCE

The National Electrical Manufacturers Association (NEMA), which represents more than 90 percent of the market for nuclear medicine imaging equipment, "is convinced of the need for larger numbers of practitioners trained in the technical acquisition, pharmaceutical manufacture, and clinical interpretation of images in nuclear medicine. This will include physicists, radiopharmacists, and clinician readers" (Richard Eaton, NEMA, personal communication). This statement is supported by a recent report that surveyed the need for nuclear medicine scientists (Center for Health Workforce Studies 2006). Based on this survey, 86 percent of 310 respon-

---

[1]Kinases are enzymes that transfer phosphate groups to other molecules.

dents in the fields of chemistry, pharmacy, physics, computer science and engineering, and other disciplines stated that very few qualified candidates were available.

8.2.1 Chemists

One of the most enriching aspects of radiopharmaceutical research is that it is generally carried out in an interdisciplinary environment where chemists work together with physicians, physicists, and biologists, sharing the excitement of solving important problems in medicine. Chemists who work in this discipline are often attracted by the opportunity to integrate chemistry with other imaging sciences, such as instrumentation. For example, the development of a new generation of small-animal imaging and multimodality imaging instruments created new challenges for the radiopharmaceutical chemist to produce radiopharmaceuticals with the very high specific activity necessary to conduct tracer studies in small animals.

Chemists who work in the field of nuclear medicine are trained in radiotracer techniques through a variety of mechanisms. Although formal radiochemistry graduate programs exist in the United States, the number has been declining because of lack of adequate funding, and there are few radiochemistry graduate programs. It is estimated that only 5 to 10 new doctoral degrees in radiochemistry are granted each year (Greg Choppin, Florida State University, personal communication). Most radiopharmaceutical chemists in the field are recruited from graduate and postgraduate university programs in organic, inorganic, medicinal, and analytical chemistry and add radiochemical skills through their postdoctoral experience. Some doctoral dissertations are written for work performed in nuclear medicine research laboratories where the principal radiopharmaceutical chemist holds an auxiliary or adjunct appointment in chemistry, nuclear/biomedical engineering, or another related field. As a result, there are few formal courses in radiochemical and radiopharmaceutical theory and practice. Moreover many if not most radiochemists are relatively specialized, concentrating on fluorine, other halogen, or technetium chemistry.

Another mechanism by which chemists from other disciplines obtain their training in radiolabeling techniques is through continuing education courses conducted by universities, scientific societies (e.g., American Chemical Society, Society of Radiopharmaceutical Sciences), the national laboratories, other Department of Energy (DOE) entities, the National Institutes of Health (NIH), or industrial training programs. Many also receive additional training on the job in the research environment. These efforts, however, lack the required depth, and these training pathways are insufficient to meet the needs of the anticipated advanced technologies that will become available in the future.

In April 2002, the DOE Office of Biological and Environmental Research held a workshop on Radiochemistry Research Resources (DOE 2002). Attending the workshop were representatives from radiopharmaceutical chemistry training programs at universities, DOE's national laboratories, and NIH. The conclusion of the workshop was that "the current shortage of radiochemist applicants was evident" and that "at their institutions there were openings currently for postdoctoral students, junior faculty members, and senior faculty members." The assembled group of experts felt that a more extensive nationwide survey was necessary. Subsequent to that workshop, data were solicited from pharmaceutical and biotech companies as well as 30 other organizations with interest in nuclear medicine. The data confirmed a serious deficiency of radiochemistry personnel possessing the skills that will be needed for future technologies in the United States (DOE 2002).

Subsequent reviews of this field by other organizations have also come to the same conclusions. The National Research Council study that reviewed the health of the U.S. chemical research community reported that although the United States still leads chemical research worldwide, its dominance in radiochemistry is being challenged (NRC 2007). Furthermore, a recent American Chemical Society symposium[2] noted the increased need for chemists with expertise in nuclear medicine with a growing requirement for chemists with additional training in radiochemistry. Similarly, a subcommittee of the DOE Biological and Environmental Research Advisory Committee (DOE 2004) noted an acute need for additional "trained chemists (including pharmaceutical chemists, organic chemists, inorganic chemists, and peptide and protein chemists) with an interest and ability in the design and synthesis of molecular imaging and targeted probes." On the basis of a survey of 20 institutions, that subcommittee reported that on average, two to three positions per institution went unfilled because of a lack of qualified applicants. The International Atomic Energy Agency (IAEA) has conducted a worldwide study of radiochemistry personnel and determined that only India and China have sufficient numbers to meet current and future needs (IAEA 2002).

The committee's own review concurs that one of the continuing challenges is to recruit new chemists. Feedback and discussions with all of our constituents revealed concerns about the lack of radiochemistry personnel at academic institutions and in industry. Industry representatives stated that there is a need for organic and medicinal chemists with strong backgrounds in radiochemistry to provide the expertise needed for drug discovery and development (personal communication, William Clarke, GE Healthcare).

---

[2] 21st Century Radiochemistry Opportunities: A Symposium Highlighting Nuclear Science Workforce Needs, March 2006, (http://oasys2.confex.com/acs/231nm/techprogram/).

8.2.2 Radiopharmacists

Closely associated with the shortage of radiochemists is the rapidly growing need for more radiopharmacists. Currently there are several ways in which pharmacists become involved in the field of nuclear medicine. They can complete advanced degrees (Ph.D. or M.S.) in radiopharmacy, take advanced courses in nuclear pharmacy following their completion of pharmacy school, or simply take the necessary training to become a Nuclear Regulatory Commission (U.S. NRC) "authorized user."[3] The Board of Pharmaceutical Specialties also provides a nuclear pharmacy specialty certification. According to the Society of Nuclear Medicine, 468 pharmacists held such certification in the United States in 2003.

With a new emphasis on research in molecular imaging at academic medical centers, the increasing expansion of commercial radiopharmaceutical companies supplying hospitals with unit doses, and the rapid expansion in commercial positron emission tomography (PET) facilities, there is considerable demand for individuals with radiopharmacy training and experience. Industry is acutely aware of this shortage since they are having difficulty filling the job openings as nuclear medicine becomes more vital in patient care. NEMA reports that there are approximately 350 commercial nuclear pharmacies in the United States with another 50 opening over the next 5 years. These pharmacies will generate the need for an additional 150 nuclear pharmacists. Industry alone will need a steady supply of approximately 200 nuclear pharmacists per year.

Currently the majority of nuclear pharmacists has received only the necessary training to become an "authorized user," which consist of 700 hours of didactic instruction in basics of radiation methods and protection. This training is most commonly obtained as part of a doctor of pharmacy degree or as a nondegree "authorized user" postgraduate course. Continuing education courses are also conducted by universities and scientific societies for pharmacists to become "authorized users."

Radiopharmacists needed to provide the necessary faculty and individuals capable of leading the research efforts required to advance the field of nuclear medicine are educated primarily in university schools of pharmacy. They receive a bachelor's degree in pharmacy and then complete additional course work in radiopharmacy or enroll in graduate M.S. or Ph.D. programs specifically in radiopharmacy. There are currently very few such

---

[3]The U.S. NRC regulates the use of radioactive material in medicine by issuing licenses to medical facilities and users. Research involving human subjects using radioactive materials may only be performed if the licensee has fulfilled the requirements outlined in 10 CFR Part 35. To become an authorized user, the applicant must complete a minimum of 700 hours of training.

programs (less than a dozen), each with a limited number of trainees. There is a critical need to expand these programs.

8.2.3 Physical Scientists and Engineers

Physicists' involvement in nuclear medicine is broad and diverse, including the disciplines of medical physics, instrumentation, computer and computational sciences, and health physics. Physicists trained in these disciplines are essential to research conducted at universities and industry, as well as in clinical practice. There are many avenues for the entry of physicists into nuclear medicine. Students with Bachelor of Science degrees or M.S. or Ph.D. degrees in physics or engineering are recruited directly into academic research institutions or industry and gain experience in such areas as imaging techniques and instrumentation, cyclotron targetry and engineering, and data processing. There are also university programs for individuals to obtain M.S. or Ph.D. degrees in subspecialty areas of medical physics, such as medical nuclear physics, diagnostic radiological physics, medical health physics, and therapeutic radiological physics. Currently, eight universities in the United States offer graduate programs in medical physics. The eight universities provide postdoctoral research programs, clinical residencies, and bioengineering programs, and all are accredited by the Commission on Accreditation of Medical Physics Education Program, Inc. (CAMPEP 2007). In addition, there are 46 nonaccredited programs at medical centers throughout the United States. The American Board of Radiology and the American Board of Medical Physicists also offer certification opportunities for medical physicists. Health physicists focus on safety issues of radiation workers and are certified by the American Board of Health Physics.

In recent years, biomedical and nuclear engineering departments, respectively, have emerged as an alternative venue for the training of physical scientists and engineers for careers in nuclear medicine. The breadth of topics covered within biomedical engineering programs currently ranges from algorithm and detector development to applying the tools of molecular biology for the intelligent design of nanotechnology-driven radionuclide carrier systems. Generally, these programs have been most effective when engineering students have the opportunity to interact with medical-school-based scientists and clinicians through participation in multidisciplinary research projects. Similarly, nuclear engineering departments offer a general curriculum that encompasses the fundamentals of nuclear science, radiation measurements, and nuclear and radiation applications in biology and medicine. Some nuclear engineering students elect to participate in research projects related to nuclear medicine, radiochemistry, radiation biology, imaging, computation modeling, or other medical applications.

However, a shortage of physicists and engineers exists in many categories: medical physics, instrumentation, computer computational sciences, and health physics. The shortage of physicists can be attributed to the declining number of training programs. For example, 20 years ago 200 to 400 health physicists were being trained each year; today the number is less than 50 (Ken Miller, Pennsylvania State University, personal communication). There are currently eight accredited programs for medical physicists in the United States with approximately 350 students in training (Paul DeLuca, University of Wisconsin, personal communication). Based on the estimated needs calculated by the American Association of Physicists in Medicine (AAPM), this number of trainees is not adequate to sustain the growth that is anticipated for the field (DeLuca 2004). Based on the membership patterns estimated by AAPM, 750 students would be needed to supply 200 new physicists per year.

8.2.4 Clinician-Scientists

There is a considerable need for appropriately trained clinician-scientists to further the development and implementation of nuclear medicine diagnostic and therapeutic tools and to act as mentors for a much needed increase in trainees. The need for an increase in the number of such individuals is a result of a belief that nuclear medicine imaging mechanisms can uniquely provide clinically relevant insights into many molecular manifestations of disease. With a rapid increase in the number of cyclotrons and radiopharmacy units proximate to PET scanners, the development of new potentially useful nuclear probes of disease will multiply. The large number of new probes to be tested for their suitability on volunteers and patients will require additional research physicians from many disciplines, including nuclear medicine specialists, radiologists, cardiologists, oncologists, and neurologists. Many will need additional training in nuclear medicine and molecular imaging techniques in order to conduct the required clinical trials. Similarly, a substantial increase in the number of new radiolabeled metabolic therapies will require clinician-scientists able to investigate their utility.

The majority of specialists who perform diagnostic nuclear medicine procedures have completed residencies in nuclear medicine approved by the Accreditation Council for Graduate Medical Education. They receive certification through the American Board of Nuclear Medicine or through approved residencies in diagnostic radiology and certification by the American Board of Radiology, sometimes also with Special Competency certification in nuclear medicine. Many board-certified radiologists who have not obtained Special Competency certification in nuclear medicine are involved in the interpretation of nuclear medicine studies, as are a number of other clinical specialists such as cardiologists and neurologists. In the case of cardiologists and neurologists, specialty professional societies and their respective certifying boards have created mechanisms whereby their member physicians do not necessarily have to complete a diagnostic radiology or nuclear medicine residency to perform and interpret nuclear medicine procedures. For example, guidelines for training in cardiovascular nuclear medicine (nuclear cardiology) have been established by the American Society of Nuclear Cardiology and the American College of Cardiology. They are part of the overall training guidelines in adult cardiovascular medicine as accepted by consensus from the Core Cardiology Training Symposium in 1994. These training guidelines have been updated to include emerging imaging technologies, such as single photon emission computed tomography/computed tomography (SPECT/CT) and PET/CT hybrid modality imaging systems, and are part of the general 3-year training in cardiovascular medicine.

Training requirements and curricula may therefore vary widely among these groups of imagers. Regarding use of unsealed sources of radioactivity, practitioners require certification by the American Board of Nuclear Medicine, the American Board of Radiology with Special Competency in Nuclear Medicine, or Radiation Oncology. In addition, the practitioner must be an authorized user and meet applicable U.S. NRC and/or Agreement State[4] requirements

The training of physicians involved in research and the clinical practice of nuclear medicine will require substantial changes with the evolution of the field. One broad division within nuclear medicine can be found between nuclear medicine physicians who are predominantly involved in diagnostic imaging and those involved in targeted radionuclide therapy. However, even within diagnostic imaging, nuclear medicine has changed considerably with the advent of combined-modality imaging. Clearly, a full interpretation of an integrated PET/CT or SPECT/CT scan requires cross-training of nuclear medical specialists in radiology. There are currently few nuclear medicine physicians or radiologists competent in fully interpreting images taken with combined modality machines. For the relatively few who are competent to do so, private practice may be so intellectually and financially rewarding that additional incentives will be needed to recruit physicians to conduct clinical research.

At present, research and clinical nuclear medicine is concentrated mainly on oncology, heart disease, and neurological disorders. Although the former two are firmly established in clinical practice, most novel neurological applications of nuclear medicine have not been translated into the

---

[4]Agreement States are those states to which the U.S. NRC has transferred some of its regulatory authority. Transfer of U.S. NRC's authority to a state is an agreement that is signed by the governor of the state and the chairman of the commission.

clinic. This, however, will change with an increased development of new PET tracers useful for the diagnosis and management of dementias and other neurodegenerative diseases as well as movement disorders.

Given this background, creation of a molecular imaging residency or fellowship, where individuals can assimilate the latest technologies into clinical practice is challenging. There is little consensus on curriculum or the topics to be covered and the complement of faculty expertise needed to teach these topics. Irrespective of these challenges, the training of nuclear medicine clinician-scientists will be different within the next 5 to10 years, and preparations must be made now in order to have an appropriate number of individuals capable of translating the latest technological innovations into clinical practice.

Without an organized effort to define the skills needed to guide clinical development of these new technologies, the field will not realize its potential. Traditional nuclear medicine, radiology, cardiology, neurology, and other specialty programs are currently not training a sufficient number of multidisciplinary imaging specialists to accomplish the desired outcome. Trainees today are not being given proper incentives to pursue an academic research career or to lead clinical trials because clinical departments preferentially reward clinical work over research.

Government agencies and the private sector must also refocus their efforts to support training programs that will generate more clinician-scientists. Imaging departments and divisions need to emphasize the importance of encouraging and supporting clinician-scientists as key participants in the process of delivering state-of-the-art health care and in advancing the area of personalized medicine. The next "PET" instrument or the next "FDG" radiotracer will not be developed unless capable clinician-scientists who understand how to conduct clinical trials are in place to translate laboratory discovery into clinical practice. Clinical trials led by experienced nuclear medicine and imaging science experts will provide young clinician-scientists with the opportunity to learn the process of conducting such trials.

Cardiologists

Cardiologists share in the clinical utilization of nuclear medicine. According to industry estimates, the number of cardiac nuclear medicine procedures performed each year in the United States exceeds 7 million (about a third of all nuclear medicine procedures) (Heinz Schelbert, University of California at Los Angeles, personal communications). These procedures contribute substantially to the detection of cardiovascular disease, to the assessment of risk for cardiac mortality and morbidity, and to the stratification of cardiac patients for optimum treatment. A substantial fraction of them are performed by cardiologists alone or in collaboration with nuclear medicine physicians or radiologists. Nuclear cardiologists together with nuclear medicine physicians account for most of the ongoing clinical research activities in cardiovascular nuclear medicine; these activities rely mostly on well-established nuclear imaging techniques

Research and development of novel radionuclide-based approaches for delineating and quantifying local molecular and cellular processes in the human cardiovascular system is urgently needed so that these new approaches can be transferred into the clinic. Yet, because of a serious shortage of qualified clinician-scientists, this area of research with its potentially considerable impact on patient care has remained underdeveloped. What is needed to overcome this impairment are nuclear medicine specialists who are well trained in basic and clinical cardiovascular sciences and research methodologies. Formal training of such individuals does not yet exist.

Oncologists

In general, medical and surgical oncologists need no special training in imaging and are satisfied to accept the interpretation of imaging studies by competent diagnosticians. On the other hand, the use of targeted radionuclide therapy requires considerable cooperation between nuclear medicine and oncology. This is particularly true for therapies given to very ill patients. Antithyroid radioiodine therapy, in most instances, is done with relatively healthy patients and can be readily handled by nuclear physicians and endocrinologists. This is not the case with other radionuclide treatments, where metabolic, targeted radionuclide therapy is added to patients already being burdened with many toxic nonradioactive drugs. A nuclear medicine physician not also trained in clinical oncology cannot handle such patients alone, and close collaboration with clinical oncologists is a prerequisite. Likewise, medical and radiation oncologists often need assistance from nuclear medicine physicians, particularly in understanding results, advantages and limitations of dosimetry, radiation protection, and radiation side effects. There are no formal cross-training programs at present and experience can only be gained by an oncologist spending time in a nuclear medicine department. The matter of proper training for oncologists in the use of radioactive materials is amplified when they are involved in research projects, where the issues of radiation dosimetry, radiation protection, and radiation side effects are considerable.

Clinical Neuroscientists

Thus far, neuronuclear medicine has had a limited impact on clinical decision making. Brain imaging is mainly used for the assessment of pathomorphology,[5] and functional magnetic resonance imaging (fMRI) is used in evaluating blood flow in both healthy and diseased brains. Although functional brain imaging started with functional PET (fPET) examinations, the radiation exposure from fPET, among other factors, has prompted a shift to the use of fMRI. However, more specific molecular-imaging-based tests using radioactive molecular probes are on the horizon and could change diagnostic imaging practice in dementias, movement disorders, and possibly demyelinating disease.[6] It is foreseeable that imaging tests developed in the future will be useful for therapeutic decision making and control of disease. Thus, there will be a greater need for interactions between neurologists, neurosurgeons, neuroradiologists, and properly trained nuclear medicine physicians. Nuclear medicine physicians specializing in brain imaging will need additional skills in the interpretation of morphological imaging examinations, while neurologists, neurosurgeons, and neuroradiologists will need to develop an understanding of tracer imaging probes and tracer kinetics in relation to morphological imaging results.

Technologists

Skilled technical personnel to conduct nuclear medicine exams are necessary in both the clinical and research settings. Yet, the number of training programs for nuclear medicine technologists had already declined prior to the emergence of PET. With the introduction of PET and PET/CT into clinical practice, the need for well-trained technologists has become even more urgent. Training of nuclear medicine technologists requires 2- or 4-year college-level course work that includes practical experience and leads to a Bachelor of Arts or Associate of Arts degree. National certification of nuclear medicine technologists is conducted by the Nuclear Medicine Technology Certification Board or the American Registry of Radiological Technologists (ARRT 2005). However, much of the earlier staff shortages, especially of technologists with qualification and certification for PET/CT hybrid systems, has now been relieved because colleges began offering 1-year training programs in nuclear medicine technology to individuals with some prior imaging experience. With the likely introduction of PET/MR hybrid systems into clinical care in the near future, the challenge may again be repeated. Some concerns, however, have been expressed by technologists about whether the one-year training pathway adequately covers the technical aspects of nuclear medicine. In nuclear medicine research (unlike

---

[5]Pathomorphology is the study of structural changes in tissues or cells resulting from abnormal conditions.

[6]Demyelinating diseases are any conditions that result in damage to the protective covering (myelin sheath) that surrounds the nerves in the brain and spinal cord.

clinical nuclear medicine), a substantial shortage of qualified technologists continues to persist. This shortage has been further exacerbated by an increasing reliance on small-animal radiotracer imaging in drug discovery and research in academic medical centers and in the biotechnology and pharmaceutical industry. Industry representatives informed the committee that the number of small-animal imaging facilities in their research has dramatically increased within the past several years without a commensurate increase in the number of trained or qualified individuals. It appears that only a few clinically trained nuclear medicine technologists participate in this area of research activity, likely due to lower financial rewards. Most small-animal imaging facilities therefore are staffed by research assistants, radiopharmacists, physicists, or biomedical engineers.

8.3 FINDINGS

From the testimony presented as well as the committee's own observations and experience, the following are considered to be impediments to the realization of an expanded work-force.

1. Shortage of Nuclear Medicine Personnel. There are shortages of both clinical and research personnel in all nuclear medicine disciplines (chemists, radiopharmacists, physicists, engineers, clinician-scientists, and technologists) with an impending "generation gap" of leadership in the field. Training, particularly of radiopharmaceutical chemists, has not kept up with current demands in universities, medical institutions, and industry, a problem that is exacerbated by a critical shortage of university faculty in nuclear chemistry and radiochemistry (NRC 2007). Nuclear medicine research requires a multidisciplinary team consisting of individuals with extremely varied education and training. Only by training an adequate number of individuals in these various disciplines will nuclear medicine and molecular imaging/therapy reach its potential. There is a pressing need for additional training programs with the proper infrastructure (including a culture of interdisciplinary science), appropriate faculty, and more doctoral students and postdoctoral fellowship opportunities.

2. Acute Shortage of Chemists. The recruitment of new chemists into the field of nuclear medicine is a significant and continual challenge. Such recruitment has been difficult because many of the chemists working in the nuclear medicine area do not have academic appointments in chemistry departments and therefore do not have access to chemistry graduate students. Thus, it is essential to reach out to chemistry students at the undergraduate and graduate student levels to fill the pipeline and avoid an impending generation gap in leadership in radiopharmaceutical chemistry. Furthermore, with the current decline in the number of U.S. students going into chemistry, the restriction of training grants to U.S. citizens and permanent residents as required by the Public Health Service Act[7] is an impediment to recruitment of new talent into the field.

8.4 RECOMMENDATIONS

RECOMMENDATION 1: *Train nuclear medicine scientists. To address the shortage of nuclear medicine scientists, engineers, and research physicians, the NIH and the DOE, in conjunction with specialty societies, should consider convening expert panels to identify the most critical national needs for training and determine how best to develop appropriate curricula to train the next generation of scientists and provide for their support.*

RECOMMENDATION 2: *Provide additional, innovative training grants. To address the needs documented in this report, specialized instruction of chemists from overseas could be accomplished in some innovative fashion (particularly in DOE-supported programs) by linking training to research. This might take the form of subsidies for course development and delivery as well as tuition subventions. By directly linking training to specific research efforts, such subventions would differ from conventional NIH/DOE training grants.*

---

[7]The Public Health Service Act restricts training awards to U.S. citizens and permanent residents. The law was implemented through the Code of Federal Regulations (http://grants1.nih.gov/training/NRSA_NameChangeLegislation.rtf) (NIH 2002).

References

ACR (American College of Radiology). 2007. Procedures per Medicare fee-for-service by imaging modality. Available from ACR Research Department.

ACRIN (American College of Radiology Imaging Network). 2007. Available at http://www.acrin.org/. Accessed February 7, 2007.

Adelstein, S. J., A. Kassis, L. Bodei, and G. Mariani. 2003. Radiotoxicity of iodine-125 and other Auger-electron-emitting radionuclides: Background to therapy. Cancer Biother Radiopharm 18:301–316.

Akabani, G., S. Carlin, P. Welch, and M. R. Zalutsky. 2006. In vitro cytotoxicity of ^{211}At-labeled trastuzumab in human breast cancer cell lines: Effect of specific activity and HER2 receptor heterogeneity on survival fraction. Nucl Med Biol 33:333–347.

Alexander, G. E., K. Chen, P. Pietrini, S. I., Rapoport, and E. M. Reiman. 2002. Longitudinal PET evaluation of cerebral metabolic decline in dementia: A potential outcome measure in Alzheimer's disease treatment studies. Am J Psychiatry 159:738–745.

AMA (American Medical Association). 2006. Report 2 of the Council on Science and Public Health (A-06) Full Text: Ionizing Radiation Exposure in the Medical Setting. Available at http://www.ama-assn.org/ama/pub/category/print/16406.html. Accessed July 18, 2007.

American Chemical Society. 2006. 21st Century Radiochemistry Opportunities: a Symposium Highlighting Nuclear Science Workforce Needs. Atlanta, GA.

Amis, E. S., Jr., P. F. Butler, K. E. Applegate, S. B. Birnbaum, L. F. Brateman, J. M. Hevezi, F. A. Mettler, R. L. Morin, M. J. Pentecost, G. G. Smith, K. J. Strauss, and R. K. Zeman. 2007. American College of Radiology white paper on radiation dose in medicine. J Am Coll Radiol 4:272–284.

Antunes, P., M. Ginj, H. Zhang, B. Waser, R. P. Baum, J. C. Reubi, and H. Maecke. 2007. Are radiogallium-labelled DOTA-conjugated somatostatin analogues superior to those labelled with other radiometals? Eur J Nucl Med Mol 34:983–993.

ARRT (The American Registry of Radiologic Technologists). 2005. Nuclear medicine technology didactic and clinical competency requirements. Available at http://www.arrt.org/education/CompReqs/NMT_CX_2005.pdf. Accessed March 29, 2007.

Badawi, R. 1999. Introduction to PET physics. Available at http://depts.washington.edu/nuc-med/IRL/pet_intro/toc.html. Accessed on February 8, 2007.

Bergen, A. W., and N. E. Caporaso. 1999. Cigarette smoking. J Natl Cancer Institute 91: 1365–1375.

Bernard, J., and L. W. Hu. 2000. University research reactors: Issues and challenges. Nuclear Tech 131:379–384.

Boyd, M., S. C. Ross, J. Dorrens, N. E. Fullerton, K. W. Tan, M. R. Zalutsky, and R. J. Mairs. 2006. Radiation-induced biologic bystander effect elicited in vitro by targeted radiopharmaceuticals labeled with α-, ß-, and auger electron–emitting radionuclides. J Nucl Med 47:1007–1015.

Brooks, D. J. 2007. Imaging non-dopaminergic function in Parkinson's disease. Mol Imaging Biol 9:217–222.

CAMPEP (Commission on Accreditation of Medical Physics Education Programs, Inc.). 2007. CAMPEP Accredited Graduate Programs in Medical Physics. Available at http://www.campep.org/campeplst.grad.asp. Accessed on May 8, 2007.

Cantana, C., Y. Wu, M. S. Judenhofer, J. Qi, B. J. Pichler, and S. R. Cherry. 2006. Simultaneous acquisition of multislice PET and MR images: Initial results with a MR-compatible PET scanner. J Nucl Med 47:1968–1976.

CDC (Centers for Disease Control and Prevention). 2006. Breast Cancer: Fast Facts. Available at http://www.cdc.gov/cancer/breast/basic_info/facts.htm. Accessed on July 26, 2007.

Center for Health Workforce Studies. 2006. Characteristic and Attitudes of Nuclear Medicine Scientists: Findings and Recommendations Based on a 2006 Survey.

Chen, P., J. Wang, K. Hope, L. Jin, J. Dick, R. Cameron, J. Brandwein, M. Minden, and R. M. Reilly. 2006. Nuclear localizing sequences promote nuclear translocation and enhance the radiotoxicity of the anti-CD33 monoclonal antibody HuM195 labeled with ^{111}In in human myeloid leukemia cells. J Nucl Med 47: 827–836.

Chen, W., T. Cloughesy, N. Kamdar, N. Satyamurthy, M. Bergsneider, L. Liau, P. Mischel, J. Czernin, M. E. Phelps, and D. H. Silverman. 2005. Imaging proliferation in brain tumors with ^{18}F-FLT-PET: Comparison with ^{18}F-FDG. J Nucl Med 46:945–952.

Chen, W., D.H. Silverman, S. Delaloye, J. Czernin, N. Kamdar, W. Pope, N. Satyamurthy, C. Schiepers, and T. Cloughesy. 2006. ^{18}F-FDOPA PET imaging of brain tumors: Comparison study with ^{18}F-FDG PET and evaluation of diagnostic accuracy. J Nucl Med 47:904–911.

Cherry, S. R. 2006. The 2006 Henry N. Wagner Lecture: Of mice and men (and positrons)—advances in PET imaging technology. J Nucl Med 47:1735–1745.

Collins, J. M., and R. L. Wahl. 2002. PET and drug R&D. Principles and Practice of Positron Emisssion Tomography. Philadelphia: Lippincott Williams & Wilkins.

Couturier, O., S. Supiot, M. Degraef-Mougin, A. Faivre-Chauvet, T. Carlier, J. F. Chatal, F. Davodeau, and M. Cherel. 2005. Cancer radioimmunotherapy with alpha-emitting nuclides. Nucl Med Mol Imaging 32:601–614.

Davies, A. J., A. Z., Rohatiner, S. Howell, K. E. Britton, S. E. Owens, I. N. Micallef, D. P. Deakin, B. M. Carrington, J. A. Lawrence, S. Vinniecombe, S. J. Mather, J. Clayton, R. Foley, H. Jan, S. Kroll, M. Harris, J. Amess, A. J. Norton, T. A. Lister, and J. A. Radford. 2004. Tositumomab and iodine I-131 tositumomab for recurrent indolent and transformed B-cell non-Hodgkin's lymphoma. J Clin Oncol 22:1469–1479.

Davila-Roman, V. G., G. Vedala, P. Herrero, L. de las Fuentes, J. G. Rogers, D. P. Kelly, and R. J. Gropler. 2002. Altered myocardial fatty acid and glucose metabolism in idiopathic dilated cardiomyopathy. J Am Coll Cardiol 40:271–277.

DeLuca, P. 2004. Education and Training for Medical Physicists: an Emergent Career Opportunity. NCI & NIBIB Young Investigator Workshop.

DeNardo, S. J. 2005. Radioimmunodetection and therapy of breast cancer. Review. Semin Nuc Med 35:143–151.

DHHS (Department of Health and Human Services). 2003. General overview of standard for privacy of individually identifiable health information. Available at http://www.hhs.gov/ocr/hipaa/guidelines/overview.pdf. Accessed March 30, 2007.

DiMasi, J. A., R. W. Hansen, and H. G. Grabowski. 2003. The price of innovation: New estimates of drug development costs. J Health Econ 22:151–185.

Dobert, N., M. Britten, B. Assmus, U. Berner, C. Menzel, R. Lehmann, N. Hamscho, V. Schachinger, S. Dimmel, A. M. Zeiher, and F. Grunwal. 2004. Transplantation of progenitor cells after reperfused acute myocardial infarction: Evaluation of perfusion and myocardial viability with FDG-PET and thallium SPECT. Eur J Nucl Med Mol Imaging 31:1146–1151.

DOE (U.S. Department of Energy). 2001. Vital Legacy of BER Medical Sciences 50-Year Commitment to Improved Healthcare through Nuclear Medicine. Available at http://doemedicalsciences.org/pubs/sc0033/vitals.html. Accessed on January 31, 2007.

DOE (U.S. Department of Energy). 2002. DOE Workshop: Radiochemistry Research Resources. Medical Sciences Division, Biological and Environmental Research, Office of Science, U.S. Department of Energy, Chicago.

DOE (U.S. Department of Energy). 2004. Radiopharmaceutical Development and the Office of Science. Report prepared by a Subcommittee of the BERAC. Available at http://www.er.doe.gov/OBER/berac/Reports.html. Accessed on February 8, 2007.

DOE (U.S. Department of Energy). 2005. Audit Report: Management of the Department's Isotope Program. DOE/IG-0709. Washington, DC: DOE.

DOE (U.S. Department of Energy). 2006. The Programs of the Office of Science. Available at http://www.science.doe.gov/grants/progdesc.html. Accessed on January 31, 2007.

DOE (U.S. Department of Energy). 2007a. ACHRE Report: The Atomic Energy Commission and Postwar BioMedical Radiation Research. Available at http://www.so.doe.gov/HealthSafety/ohre/roadmap/achre/intro_4.html. Accessed on August 6, 2007.

DOE (U.S. Department of Energy). 2007b. Office of Biological & Environmental Research: Medical Services Division. Available at http://www.science.doe.gov/ober/msd_top.html. Accessed on February 8, 2007.

Du, Y., J. Honeychurch, M. S. Cragg, M. J. Glennie, P. W. Johnson, and T. M. Illidge. 2004. Antibody-induced intracellular signaling works in combination with radiation to eradicate lymphoma in radioimmunotherapy. Blood 103:1485–1494.

Dunphy, M. P., A. Freidman, S. M. Larson, and H. W. Strauss. 2005. Association of vascular ^{18}F-FDG uptake with vascular calcification. J Nucl Med 46:1278–84.

Eckelman, W. C. 2003.The use of PET and knockout mice in the drug discovery process. Drug Discovery Today 8:404–410.

Eckelman, W. C., and P. Richards. 1970. Instant 99m-Tc-DTPA. J Nucl Med 11:761.

Eckelman, W. C., and P. Richards. 1971. Instant 99m-Tc compounds. J Nucl Med 10:245–251.

Engler, H., A. Forsberg, O. Almkvist, G. Blomquist, E. Larsson, I. Savitcheva, A. Wall, A. Ringheim, B. Langstrom, and A. Nordberg. 2006. Two-year follow-up of amyloid deposition in patients with Alzheimer's disease. Brain 129:2856–2866.

Enns, L., K. T. Bogen, J. Wizniak, A. D. Murtha, and M. Meinfeld. 2004. Low-dose radiation hypersensitivity is associated with p53-dependent apoptosis. Mol Cancer Res 2:557–566.

Erondu, N., I. Gantz, B. Musser, S. Survawanshi, M. Mallick, C. Addy, J. Cote, G. Bray, K. Fujioka, H. Bays, P. Hollander, S. M. Sanabrai-Bohorquez, W. Eng, B. Langstrom, R. J. Hargreaves, H. D. Burns, A. Kanatani, T. Fukami, D. J. MacNeil, K. M. Gottesdiener, J. M. Amatruda, K. D. Kaufman, and S. B. Heymsfield. 2006. Neuropeptide Y5 receptor antagonism does not induce clinically meaningful weight loss in overweight and obese adults. Cell Metab 4: 275–282.

FDA (U.S. Food and Drug Administration). 2005. Guidance for Industry INDS: Approaches to Complying with CGMP During Phase I. Available at www.fda.gov/cber/gdlns/indcgmp.htm. Accessed on May 10, 2007.

FDA (U.S. Food and Drug Administration). 2006a. Guidance for Industry, Investigation, and Reviewers Exploratory IND Studies. Available at http://www.fda.gov/CDER/guidance/7086fnl.pdf. Accessed on February 8, 2007.

FDA (U.S. Food and Drug Administration). 2006b. Memorandum of Understanding between the FDA and the National Cancer Institute and the Centers for Medicaid and Medicare Services. MOU No. 225-06-8001.

FDA (U.S. Food and Drug Administration). 2007. Listing of Approved Oncology Drugs with Approved Indications. Available at http://www.fda.gov/cder/cancer/druglistframe.htm. Accessed on February 8, 2007.

Fowler, J. S., and T. Ido. 2002. Initial and subsequent approach for the synthesis of ^{18}F-FDG. Semin Nuc Med 32:6–12.

Fowler, J. S., Y. S. Ding, and N. D. Volkow. 2003. Radiotracers for positron emission tomography. Seminars in Nuclear Medicine 33:14–27.

Garber, K. 2004. Energy boost: The Warburg effect returns in a new theory of cancer. J Natl Cancer Institute 96:1805–1806.

Gokhale, A. S., J. Mayadev, B. Pohlman, and R. M. Macklis. 2005. Gamma camera scans and pretreatment tumor volumes as predictors of response and progression after Y-90 anti-CD20 radioimmunotherapy. Int J Radiat Oncol Biol Phys 63:194–201.

Goldenberg, D. M., R. M. Sharkey, G. Paganelli, J. Barbet, and J. F. Chatal. 2006. Antibody pretargeting advances cancer radioimmunodetection and radioimmunotherapy. J Clin Oncol 24:823–834.

Herceptin. 2007. HER2 positive metastatic breast cancer treatment. Available at http://www.herceptin.com/herceptin. Accessed June 18, 2007.

IAEA (International Atomic Energy Agency). 2002. Assessment of the Teaching and Applications in Radiochemistry.

IOM (Institute of Medicine). 1995. Isotopes for Medicine and the Life Sciences, S. J. Adelstein and J. F. Manning, eds. Washington, DC: National Academy Press.

Juweid, M. E. and B. D. Cheson. 2006. Positron emission tomography and assessment of cancer therapy. N Engl J Med 354:496–507.

Karp, J. S. 2006. Time-of-flight PET. PET Center of Excellence Newsletter.

Kates, A. M., P. Herrero, C. Dence, P. Soto, M. Srinivasan, D. G. Delano, A. Ahsani, and R. J. Gropler. 2003. Impact of aging on substrate metabolism by the human heart. J Am Coll Cardiol 41:293–299.

Kelloff, G. J., J. M. Hoffman, B. Johnson, H. I. Scher, B. A. Siegel, E. Y. Cheng, B. D. Cheson, J. O'Shaughnessy, K. Z. Guyton, D. A. Mankoff, L. Shankar, S. M. Larson, C. C. Sigman, R. L. Schilsky, and D. C. Sullivan. 2005. Progress and promise of FDG-PET imaging for cancer patient management and oncologic drug development. Clin Cancer Res 11:2785–2808.

Ketchum, L. E., M. A. Green, and S. S. Jurisson. 1997. Research radionuclide availability in North America. J Nucl Med 38:15N–19N.

Klunk, W. E., H. Engler, A. Nordberg , Y. Wang, G. Blomqvist, D. P. Holt, M. Bergstrom, I. Savitcheva, G. F. Huand, S. Estrada, B. Ausen, M. L. Debnath, J. Barletta, J. C. Price, J. Sandell, B. J. Lopresti, A. Wall, P. Koivisto, G. Antoni, C. A. Mathis, and B. Langstrom. 2004. Imaging brain amyloid in Alzheimer's disease with Pittsburgh Compound-B. Ann Neurol 55:306–319.

Koob, G. F. 2006. The neurobiology of addiction: a neuroadaptational view relevant to diagnosis. Addiction 101(Suppl 1):23–30.

Koppe, M. J., T. Hendriks, O. C. Boerman, W. J. G. Oyen, and R. P. Bleichrodt. 2006. Radioimmunotherpay is an effective adjuvant treatment after cytoreductive surgery of experimental colonic peritoneal carcinomatosis. J Nucl Med 47:1867–1874.

Kung, H. F., M. P. Kung, and S. R. Choi. 2003. Radiopharmaceuticals for single photon emission computed tomography brain imaging. Semin Nucl Med 33:2–13.

Kwekkeboom, D. J., J. Mueller-Brand, G. Paganelli, L. B. Anthony, S. Pauwels, L. K. Kvols, T. M. O'Dorisio, R. Valkema, L. Bodei, M. Chinol, H. R. Maecke, and E. P. Krenning. 2005. Overview of results of peptide receptor radionuclide therapy with three radiolabeled somatostatin analogs. J Nucl Med 46:62S–66S.

Lardinois, D., W. Weder, T. F. Hany, E. M. Kamel, S. Korom, B. Seifert, G. K. von Schulthess, and H. C. Steinhert. 2003. Staging of non-small-cell lung cancer with integrated positron emission tomography and computed tomography. N Engl J Med 348:2500–2507.

Lee, C. C., G. Sui, A. Elizarov, C. J. Shu, Y. S. Shin, A. N. Dooley, J. Huang, A. Daridon, P. Wyatt, D. Stout, H. C. Kolb, O. N. Witte, N. Satyamurthy, J. R. Heath, M. E. Phelps, S. R. Quake, and H. R. Tseng. 2005. Multistep synthesis of a radiolabeled imaging probe using integrated microfluidics. Science 310:1793–1796.

Leyton, J., J. R. Latigo, M. Perumal, H. Dhaliwal, Q. He, and E. O. Aboagye. 2005. Early detection of tumor response to chemotherapy by 3'-deoxy-3'-[18F]fluorothymidine positron emission tomography: The effect of cisplatin on a fibrosarcoma tumor model in vivo. Cancer Res 65:4202–4210.

Liersch, T., J. Meller, B. Kulle, T. M. Behr, P. Markus, C. Langer, B. M. Ghadimi, W. A. Wegener, J. Kovacs, I. D. Horak, H. Becker, and D. M. Goldenberg. 2005. Phase II trial of carcinoembroynic antigen radioimmunotherapy with ^{131}I-labetuzumab after salvage resection of colorectal metastases in the liver: 5-year safety and efficacy results. J Clin Oncol 23:6763–6770.

Macklis, R. M. 2004. How and why does radioimmunotherapy work? Int J Radiat Oncol Biol Phys 59:1269–1271.

Madsen M. T., J. A. Anderson, J. R. Halama, J. Kleck, D. J. Simpkin, J. R. Votaw, R. E. Wendt, L. E. Williams, and M. V. Yester. 2006. AAPM Task Group 108: PET and PET/CT shielding requirements. Med Phys 33:4–15.

Mairs, R. J., S. H. Cunningham, M. Boyd, and S. Carlin. 2000. Applications of gene transfer to targeted radiotherapy. Current Pharm Design 14:1419–1432.

Matthay, K. K., J. C. Tan, J. G. Villablanca, G. A. Yanik, J. Veatch, B. Franc, E. Twomey, B. Horn, C. P. Reynolds, S. Groshen, R. C. Seeger, and J. M. Maris. 2006. Phase I dose escalation of iodine-131-metaiodobenzylguanidine with myeloablative chemotherapy and autologous stem-cell transplantation in refractory neuroblastoma: New approaches to Neuroblastoma Therapy Consortium Study. J Clin Oncol 24:500–506.

Mothersill, C., and C. B. Seymour. 2004. Radiation-induced bystander effects—implications for cancer. Nature Reviews Cancer 4:158–164.

Mottram, J.C. 1936. Factor of importance in radiosensitivity of tumors. Br J Radio 9:606.

Mullin, R. 2003. Drug development costs about $1.7 billion. Chem Eng News 81:8.

Myers, R., and S. Hume. 2002. Small animal PET. Eur Neuropsychopharmacol 12:545–555.

Namdar, M., T. F. Hany, P. Koepfli, P. T. Siegrist, C. Burger, C. A. Wyss, T. F. Luscher, G. K. von Schulthess, and P. A. Kaufmann. 2005. Integrated PET/CT for the assessment of coronary artery disease: A feasible study. J Nucl Med. 46:930–935

Nariai T., Y. Tanaka, H. Wakimoto, M. Aoyagi, M. Tamaki, K. Ishiwata, M. Senda, K. Ishii, K. Hirakawa, and K. Ohno. 2005. Usefulness of L-[methyl-11C]methionine-positron emission tomography as a biological monitoring tool in the treatment of glioma. J Neurosurg 103:498–507.

NCI (National Cancer Institute). 2005. Understand Cancer Series: Molecular Diagnostics. Available at http://www.cancer.gov/cancertopics/understandingcancer/moleculardiagnostics. Accessed February 8, 2007.

NCI (National Cancer Institute). 2007a. The Cancer Genome Atlas Project website. Available at http://cgap.nci.nih.gov/. Accessed on February 8, 2007.

NCI (National Cancer Institute). 2007b. Cancer Imaging Program. Available at http://imaging.cancer.gov/programsandresources/specializedinitiatives/dcide. Accessed on February 8, 2007.

NCRP (National Council on Radiation Protection and Measurements). 1991. Commentary No. 7: Misadministration of radioactive material in medicine—scientific background.

NCRP (National Council on Radiation Protection and Measurements). 2007. 43rd Annual Meeting—Advances in Radiation Protection in Medicine.

NIA (National Institute on Aging). July 2006. Fact Sheet. NIH Publication No. 06-3431. Available at http://www.alzheimers.nia.nih.gov. Accessed on February 8, 2007.

Nicolini, M., and U. Mazzi. 1999. Editorial. Technetium, rhenium and other metals in chemistry and nuclear medicine, Padova, Italy.

NIH (National Institutes of Health). 2002. Title 42. The Public Health Service National Research Institutes Awards and Training. Available at http://grants1.nih.gov/training/NRSA_NameChangeLegislation.rtf. Accessed on May 8, 2007.

NIH (National Institutes of Health). 2006. Information on Clinical Trials and Human Research Studies. Available at http://www.ClinicalTrials.gov. Accessed on February 8, 2007.

Nilsson, S., R.H. Larsen, S.D. Foss, L. Balteskard, K.W. Borch, J.E. Westlin, G. Salberg, and Y.S. Bruland. 2005. First clinical experience with α-emitting radium-223 in the treatment of skeletal metastases. Clin Cancer Res 11:4451–4459.

NIMH (National Institute of Mental Health). 2006. Obesity Linked with Mood and Anxiety Disorders. Available at http://www.nimh.nig.gov/press/obesity_mooddisorders.cfm. Accessed on February 8, 2007.

NLM (National Library of Medicine). 1998. HSTAT Health Services/Technology Assessment Text: Cost of PET. Available at http://www.ncbi.nlm.nih.gov/books/bv.fcgi?rid=hstat6.section.2250. Accessed on February 8, 2007.

NINDS (National Institute of Neurological Disorders and Stroke). 2006a. Frontotemporal Dementia Information Page. Available at http://www.ninds.nih.gov/disorders/picks/picks.htm?css=print. Accessed on February 8, 2007.

NINDS (National Institute of Neurological Disorders and Stroke). 2006b. Huntington Disease. Available at http://www.ninds.nih.gov/disorders/huntington/huntington.htm. Accessed on January 8, 2007.

NNI (National Nanotechnology Initiative). 2007. Applications/Products. Available at http://www.nano.gov/html/facts/appsprod.html. Accessed on February 8, 2007.

NRC (National Research Council). 1982. Separated Isotopes: Vital Tools for Science & Medicine. Washington, DC: National Academy Press.

NRC (National Research Council). 2006. Health Risks from Exposure to Low Levels of Ionizing Radiation: BEIR VII Phase 2. National Research Council. Washington, DC: The National Academies Press.

NRC (National Research Council). 2007. Benchmarking the Research Competitiveness of the United States in Chemistry. Washington, DC: The National Academies Press.

Nuclear Energy Agency. 2000. Beneficial Uses and Production of Isotopes, 2000 update.

Nunn, A. D. 2006. The cost of developing imaging agents for routine clinical use. Investigative Radiol 41:206–212.

O'Donoghue, J. A., G. Sgouros, C. R. Divgi, and J. L. Humm. 2000. Single-dose versus fractionated radioimmunotherapy: model comparisons for uniform tumor dosimetry. J Nucl Med 41:538–547.

O'Shaughnessy, J. A. 2006. Molecular signatures predict outcomes of breast cancer. N Engl J Med 355:615–617.

Palmer, S.E. 1999. Vision Science: Photons to Phenomenology. Cambridge, MA: MIT Press.

Phelps, Michael. 2006. Presentation to the Committee on State of Science of Nuclear Medicine, San Francisco, CA. November 15.

PHRMA. 2006. 2006 Report: Medicines in development for cancer. Available at http://newmeds.phrma.org/. Accessed on February 8, 2007.

Piccart-Gebhard, M. J., M. Procter, B. Leyland-Jones, A. Goldhirsch, M. Untch, I. Smith, L. Gianni, J. Baselga, R. Bell, C. Jackisch, D. Cameron, M. Dowsett, C. H. Barrios, G. Steger, C. S. Huang, M. Andersson, M. Inbar, M. Lichinitser, I. Lang, U. Nitz, H. Iwata, C. Thomssen, C. Lohrisch, T. M. Suter, J. Ruschoff, T. Suto, V. Greatorex, C. Ward, C. Straehle, E. McFadden, M. S. Dolci, R. D., Gelber, and Herceptin Adjuvant (HERA) Trial Study Team. 2005. Trastuzumab after adjuvant chemotherapy in HER2-positive breast cancer. N Engl J Med 353:1659–1672.

Piccini, P., and A. Whone. 2004. Functional brain imaging in the differential diagnosis of Parkinson's disease. Lancet Neurol 3:284–290.

Pirotte, B., S. Goldman, N. Massager, P. David, D. Wikler, A. Vandesteene, I. Salmon, J. Brotchi, and M. Levivier. 2004. Comparison of ^{18}F-FDG and ^{11}C-methionine for PET-guided stereotactic brain biopsy of gliomas. J Nucl Med 45:1293–1298.

Pohlman, B. L., J. W. Sweetenham, and R. M. Macklis. 2006. Review of clinical radioimmunotherapy. Expert Rev Anticancer Ther 6: 445–461.

Press, O. W. 2003. Radioimmunotherapy for non-Hodgkin's lymphomas: A historical perspective. Semin Oncol 30(2 Suppl 4):10–21.

Rajendran J. G., K. R. Hendrickson, A. M. Spence, M. Muzi, K. A. Krohn, and D. A. Mankoff. 2006. Hypoxia imaging-directed radiation treatment planning. Eur J Nucl Med Mol Imaging. 33:44–53.

Reardon, D. A., G. Akabani, R. E. Coleman, A. H. Friedman, H. S. Friedman, J. E. Herndon, R. E. McLendon, C. N. Pegram, J. M. Provenzale, J. A. Quinn, J. N. Rich, J. Vredenburgh, A. Desjardins, S. Guruangan, M. Badruddoja, J. Dowell, T. Z. Wong, X. G. Zhao, M. R. Zalutsky, and D. D. Bigner. 2006. Salvage radioimmunotherapy with murine ^{131}I-labeled anti-tenascin monoclonal antibody 81C6 for patients with recurrent primary and metastatic malignant brain tumors: Phase II study results. J Clin Oncol 24:115–122.

Reba, R. C., R. W. Atcher, R. G. Bennett, R. D. Finn, L. C. Knight, H. H. Kramer, S. Mtingwa, T. J. Ruth, D. C. Sullivan, and J. B. Woodward. 2000. Final Report. NERAC Subcommittee for Isotope Research & Production Planning, pp 1–32. Available at http://www.nuclear.gov/nerac/finalisotopereport.pdf. Accessed on February 8, 2007.

Rivarda, M. J., L. M. Bobekb, R. A. Butlerc, M. A. Garlandd, D. J. Hille, J. K. Kriegerf, J. B. Muckerheideg, B. D. Pattone, and E. B. Silberstein. 2005. The U.S. national isotope program: Current status and strategy for future success. Appl Radiat Isot 63:157–178.

Rogers, K. C. 2002. The past and future of university research reactors. Science 295: 2217–2218.

Schoenhagen, P., S. S. Halliburton, A. E. Stillman, S. A. Kuzmiak, S. E. Nissen, E. M. Tuzcu, and R. D. White. 2004. Noninvasive imaging of coronary arteries: Current and future role of multi-detector row CT. Radiology 232:7–17.

Sequist, L. V., D. W. Bell, T. J. Lynch, and D. A. Haber. 2007. Molecular predictors of response to epidermal growth factor receptor antagonists in non-small-cell lung cancer. J Clin Oncol 25:587–595.

Sharkey, R. M., and D. M. Goldenberg. 2005. Perspectives on cancer therapy with radiolabeled monoclonal antibodies. J Nucl Med 46:115S–127S.

Shields, A. F. 2006. Positron emission tomography measurement of tumor metabolism and growth: its expanding role in oncology. Mol Imaging Biol 8:141–150.

Shields, A. F. 2006. Positron emission tomography measurement of tumor metabolism and growth: its expanding role in oncology. Mol Imaging Biol 8:141–150.

Shields, A. F., J. R. Grierson, B. M. Dohmen, H. J. Machulla, J. C. Stayanoff, J. M. Lawhorn-Crews, J. E. Obradovich, O. Muzik, and T. J. Managner. 1998. Imaging proliferation in vivo with [F-18]FLT and positron emission tomography. Nat Med 4:1334–1336.

Silverman, D. H., G. W. Small, C. Y. Chang, C. S. Lu, M. A. Kung de Aburto, W. Chen, J. Czernin, S. I. Rapoport, P. Pietrini, G. E. Alexander, M. B. Schapiro, W. J. Jagust, J. M. Hoffman, K. A. Welsh-Bohmer, A. Alavi, C. M. Clark, E. Salmon, M. J. de Leon, R. Mielke, J. L. Cummings, A. P. Kowell, S. S. Gambhir, C. K. Hoh, and M. E. Phelps. 2001. Positron emission tomography in evaluation of dementia: Regional brain metabolism and long-term outcome. JAMA 286:2120–2127.

Spicer, K. M., S. Baron, G. D. Frey, H. O'Brien, R. C. Gostic, R. W. Rowe, and R. M. N. Spellman, eds. 1998. Proceedings of the Medical Isotope Workshop, University of South Carolina, Charleston, SC.

Small, G. W., L. M. Ercoli, D. H. Silverman, S. C. Huang, S. Komo, S. Y. Bookheimer, H. Lavretsky, K. Miller, P. Siddarth, N. L. Rasgon, J. C. Mazziotta, S. Saxena, H. M. Wu, M. S. Mega, J. L. Cummings, A. M. Saunders, M. A. Pericak-Vance, A. D. Roses, J. R. Barrio, and M. E. Phelps. 2006. Cerebral metabolic and cognitive decline in persons at genetic risk for Alzheimer's disease. Proc Natl Acad Sci U S A 97:6037–6042.

SNM (Society of Nuclear Medicine). 2005. National Radionuclide Production Enhancement (NRPE) Program: Meeting Our Nation's Need for Radionuclides.

Stanford Linear Accelerator Center. 2006. Accelerator Form and Function. Available at http://www2.slac.stanford.edu/vvc/accelerator.html. Accessed on July 6, 2007.

Taharan, N., H. Kai, M. Ishibashi, H. Nakaura, H. Kaida, K. Baba, N. Hayabuchi, and T. Imaizumi. 2006. Simvastatin attenuates plaque inflammation: evaluation by fluorodeoxyglucose positron emission tomography. J Am Coll Cardiol 48:1825–1831.

Tang, H. R., A. J. Da Silva, K. K. Matthay, D. C. Price, J. P. Huberty, R. A. Hawkins, and B. H. Hasegawa. 2001.Neuroblastoma imaging using a combined CT scanner-scintillation camera and ^{131}I-MIBG. J Nucl Med. 42:237–247.

Tawakol, A., R. Q. Migrino, G. G. Bashian, S. Bedri, D. Vermylen, R. C. Cury, D. Yates, G. M. LaMuraglia, K. Furie, S. Houser, H. Gewirtz, J. E. Muller, T. J. Brady, and A. J. Fischman. 2006. In vivo ^{18}F-fluorodeoxyglucose positron emission tomography imaging provides a noninvasive measure of carotid plaque inflammation in patients. J Am Coll Cardiol 48:1818–1824.

Tillisch, J., R. Brunken, R. Marshall, M. Schwaiger, M. Mandelkern, M. Phelps, and H. Schelbert. 1986. Reversibility of cardiac wall-motion abnormalities predicted by positron tomography. N Engl J Med 314:884–888.

Udelson J. E. and E. J. Spiegler. 2001. Emergency department perfusion imaging for suspected coronary artery disease: The ERASE Chest Pain Trial. Md Med Spring (Suppl):90–94.

University of Arkansas. For Medical Sciences Radiopharmacuetical List and Package Inserts. Available at http://nuclearpharmacy.uams.edu/resources/PackageInserts.asp. Accessed on May 7, 2007.

Wagner, H. N., R. C. Reba, R. Brown, E. Coleman, L. Knight, D. Sullivan, R. Caretta, J. W. Babich, A. Carpenter, D. Nichols, K. Spicer, S. Scott, and T. Tenforde. 1999. Expert Panel Forecast of Future Demand for Medical Isotopes. Available at http://www.ne.doe.gov/nerac/isotopedemand.pdf. Accessed on February 8, 2007.

Webber, W. A. 2005. PET for response assessment in oncology: radiotherapy and chemotherapy. Newsline. J Nucl Med 28(Suppl):42–49.

Weber, W. A., and H. Wieder. 2006. Monitoring chemotherapy and radiotherapy of solid tumors. Eur J Nucl Med Mol Imaging 33: 27–37.

Weissleder, R. 2006. Molecular Imaging in Cancer. Science 312:1168–1171.

Wieder, H. A., A. J. Beer, K. Lordick, K. Ott, M. Fischer, E.J. Rummeny, S. Ziegler, J.R. Siewer, M. Schwaiger, and W.A. Weber. 2005. Comparison of changes in tumor metabolic activity and tumor size during chemotherapy of adenocarcinomas of the esophagogastric junction. J Nucl Med 46:2029–2034.

Wierenga, D. E., and C. R. Eaton. 2007. Phases of Product Development. Office of Research and Development, Pharmaceutical Manufacturers Association.

Wiseman, G. A., E. Kornmehl, B. Leigh, W. D. Erwin, D. A. Podoloff, S. Spies, R. B. Sparks, M. G. Stabin, T. Witzig, and C. A. White. 2003. Radiation dosimetry results and safety correlations from ^{90}Y-ibritumomab tiuxetan radioimmunotherapy for relapsed or refractory non-Hodgkin's Lymphoma. J Nucl Med 44:465–474.

Witzig, T. E., L. I. Gordon, F. Cabanillas, M. S. Czuczman, C. Emmanouilides, R. Joyce, B. L. Pohlman, N. L. Bartlett, G. A. Wiseman, N. Padre, A. J. Grillo-Lopez, P. Multani, and C. A. White. 2002. Randomized controlled trial of yttrium-90-labeled ibritumomab tiuxetan radioimmunotherapy versus rituximab immunotherapy for patients with relapsed or refractory low-grade, follicular, or transformed B-cell non-Hodgkin's lymphoma. J Clin Oncol 20:2453–2463.

Zalutsky, M. R. 2003. Radionuclide therapy. Pp 315–348 in *Handbook of Nuclear Chemistry Volume 4: Radiochemistry and Radiopharmaceutical Chemistry in Life Sciences.* Roesch, F., ed. Dordrecht, Netherlands: Kluwer Academic.

Zasadny, K. R., and R. L. Wahl. 1993. Standardized uptake values of normal tissues at PET with 2-[fluorine-18]-fluoro-2-deoxy-D-glucose: variations with body weight and a method for correction. Radiology 189:846–850.

Zipursky, R. B., J. H. Meyer, and N. P. Verhoeff. 2007. PET and SPECT imaging in psychiatric disorders. Can J Psychiatry 52:146–157.

Appendix A

Information-Gathering Sessions

The committee organized several meetings to obtain information about the state of the science of nuclear medicine. The committee held five data-gathering sessions open to the public to receive briefings from technical experts, federal agencies, and other interested parties. The written materials (e.g., PowerPoint presentations and written statements) obtained by the committee at these open sessions are posted on the Web site for this project: http://www8.nationalacademies.org/cp/projectview.aspx?key=48654.

A.1 FIRST MEETING, JUNE 12–13, 2006, WASHINGTON, D.C.

The objective of this meeting was to obtain background information on the study request. The committee was briefed by both sponsors, the Department of Energy (DOE) and the National Institutes of Health (NIH), and by five professional organizations with an interest in nuclear medicine. The following is the list of topics and speakers for the open session:

- Mission of DOE's Isotope Program, John Pantaleo, M.S., Program Director, Isotope Programs, Office of Nuclear Energy, DOE
- DOE Support of Nuclear Medicine Research, Michael Viola, M.D., Director, Life and Medical Sciences Division, Biological and Environmental Research, Office of Science, DOE
- NIH and National Cancer Institute (NCI) Perspectives on Nuclear Medicine Research, Daniel Sullivan, M.D., Cancer Imaging Program, NCI, NIH

- National Institute of Biomedical Imaging and Bioengineering (NIBIB) Perspective on the National Academies "State of the Science in Nuclear Medicine" Study, William Heetderks, M.D., Associate Director for Extramural Science Programs, NIBIB, NIH
- Presentation to NAS Committee on "State of the Science in Nuclear Medicine," Michael Welch, Ph.D., Professor of Radiology, Washington University School of Medicine, on behalf of the Society of Nuclear Medicine
- Society of Radiopharmaceutical Sciences, William Eckelman, Ph.D., Adjunct Professor of Radiology, University of California at San Diego, on behalf of the Society of Radiopharmaceutical Sciences
- State of the Science in Nuclear Medicine: IEEE Perspective, William Moses, Ph.D., Senior Staff Scientist in the Life Sciences Division at Lawrence Berkeley National Laboratory, on behalf of the IEEE Nuclear & Plasma Sciences Society
- Issues Affecting the Future of Nuclear Medicine, Roy Brown, Senior Director, Federal Affairs, Council on Radionuclides and Radiopharmaceuticals
- Perspectives from the Society of Molecular Imaging, Thomas Budinger, M.D., Ph.D., Professor of Radiology, University of California at San Francisco, on behalf of the Society of Molecular Imaging
- State of the Science in Nuclear Medicine: A Physician-Scientist's Perspective, Richard Wahl, M.D., Henry N. Wagner, Jr., Professor of Nuclear Medicine, Johns Hopkins University, on behalf of the Academy of Radiology Research

A.2 SECOND MEETING, AUGUST 24–25, 2006, WASHINGTON, D.C.

The objective of the second meeting was to gather information on the state of the science in radiopharmaceuticals and issues surrounding isotope availability to the nuclear medicine community (charges 1 and 3 of the statement of task). The following is the list of topics and speakers who presented during the open session:

- NCI's Current and Future Commitment to Translational Research: an Interim Report of the Translational Research Working Group, Ernest Hawk, M.D., M.P.H., Director of the Office of Centers, Training, & Resources in the Office of the Director, NCI, NIH
- Radiopharmaceutical Chemistry: Future Needs and Directions, Michael Welch, Ph.D., Professor of Radiology, Molecular Biology and Pharmacology, and Biomedical Engineering, and Co-Director of the Division of Radiological Sciences, Washington University Medical School

• Supporting the Nation's Nuclear Medicine Research, Ralph Butler, M.S., Director, and Alan Ketring, Ph.D., Associate Director of the Radiopharmaceutical R&D Program, University of Missouri Research Reactor
• Radiolabeled Therapeutic Monoclonal Antibodies, Martin Brechbiel, Ph.D., Chief of the Radioimmune and Inorganic Chemistry Section, NCI, NIH
• Future Needs for Radiopharmaceutical Development for the Diagnosis and Treatment of Human Disease, Hank Kung, Ph.D., Professor of Radiology and Pharmacology, University of Pennsylvania
• National Academies' Meeting: Committee on State of the Science of Nuclear Medicine, Cynthia Flannery, M.S., Team Leader of the Medical Radiation Safety Team, Nuclear Regulatory Commission

A.3 THIRD MEETING, OCTOBER 16-17, 2006, IRVINE, CALIFORNIA

The objective of the third meeting was to gather information on issues surrounding training of personnel in nuclear medicine (charge 4). The following is the list of panelists for the open session:

• Paul DeLuca, Ph.D., Associate Dean for Research & Graduate Studies, University of Wisconsin
• Claude Meares, Ph.D., Professor of Chemistry, University of California at Davis
• Mark Green, Ph.D., Professor and Head of the Division of Nuclear Pharmacy Department of Industrial and Physical Pharmacy, School of Pharmacy and Pharmaceutical Sciences Purdue University
• Greggory Choppin, Ph.D., Senior Scientist & Project Director, Florida State University
• Jeffrey Norenberg, Ph.D., Associate Director, New Mexico Center for Isotopes in Medicine, University of New Mexico
• Michael Graham, M.D., Ph.D., Professor, Department of Radiology, University of Iowa, for American College of Radiology
• Ken Miller, M.S., Professor of Radiology & Director in Medicine, Pennsylvania State University, for Health Physics Society
• Sabee Molloi, Ph.D., Professor, Radiological Sciences, University of California at Irvine, for American Association of Physicists in Medicine
• William Jagust, M.D., Professor of Neurology, University of California at Berkeley, for American Academy of Neurology
• Ward Digby, Ph.D., Director, Siemens
• Ludger Dinkelborg, Ph.D., Head of PET Research, Schering AG
• Bernard Fine, M.D., Ph.D., Genentech

A.4 FOURTH MEETING, NOVEMBER 16–17, 2006, SAN FRANCISCO, CALIFORNIA

The objective of the fourth meeting was to gather information on future needs, instrumentation and computational needs (charge 2), targeted radionuclide therapy, and future technologies applicable to nuclear medicine. The following is the list of speakers for the open session:

• Imaging in the Brain Sciences 2006,Marcus Raichle, M.D., Professor of Radiology, Neurology, Neurobiology, Biomedical Engineering and Psychology and co-Director, Division of Radiological Sciences, Washington University School of Medicine

• State of the Science in Nuclear Medicine, Markus Schwaiger, M.D., Professor & Director, Department of Nuclear Medicine, Technical University of Munich

• Need a New Discovery Pathway for Molecular Imaging Bio and Surrogate Markers, Michael Phelps, M.D., Ph.D., Chair of Department of Molecular and Medical Pharmacology, Director of Crump Institute for Molecular Imaging, and Director of the Institute of Molecular Medicine, University of California at Los Angeles

• The Future of Nuclear Medicine at the DOE Laboratories, Stephen Derenzo, Ph.D., Senior Staff Scientist, Lawrence Berkeley National Laboratory

• SPECT and SPECT/CT Instrumentation and Computation, Bruce Hasegawa, Ph.D., Professor of Radiology, University of California at San Francisco

• Nuclear Medicine Preclinical Instrumentation Technologies: microPET and Beyond, Arion Chatziioannou, Ph.D., Assistant Professor, Department of Molecular & Medical Pharamacology, University of California at Los Angeles

• Instrumentation and Computation: Role of Modeling and Computation in Nuclear Medicine, Sung-Cheng Huang, Ph.D., Professor, Department of Molecular & Medical Pharamacology and Department of Biomathematics, University of California at Los Angeles

• Siemens Molecular Imaging, Bernard Bendriem, Ph.D., Vice President, Science & Technology, Siemens

• Susan Knox, M.D., Associate Professor, Department of Radiation Oncology, Stanford University

• David Goldenberg, M.D., Sc.D., President, Garden State Cancer Center

• Mark Kaminski, M.D., Professor, Department of Internal Medicine, Director of the Leukemia/Lymphoma Program, University of Michigan

• Alexander McEwan, M.D., Nuclear Medicine Physician and Director of Oncologic Imaging at Cross Cancer Institute, and Director of Division of Oncologic Imaging, Department of Oncology, University of Alberta

- Andrew Raubitschek, M.D., Chair, City of Hope National Medical Center
- Peter Carroll, M.D., Co-Director of Urologic Oncology Service, and Chair of Urology Department, University of California at San Francisco
- Keith McCormick, M.B.A., Senior Manager, Oncology Marketing, Biogen-IDEC
- Combining In Vitro and In Vivo Diagnostics via a Systems Biology Foundation, James Heath, Ph.D., Professor of Chemistry, California Institute of Technology
- Micro- and Nanotechnologies for Accelerated Access to Biological Information, Michael Ramsey, Ph.D., Minnie N. Goldby Distinguished Professor of Chemistry Chair, University of North Carolina
- Biological Large Scale Integration, Stephen Quake, Ph.D., Professor of Bioengineering, Stanford University

A.5 FIFTH MEETING, JANUARY 6–7, 2007, WASHINGTON, D.C.

The objective of the fifth meeting was to gather information on further sponsor perspective and regulatory hurdles facing the field of nuclear medicine. The following is the list of speakers for the open session:

- Michael Viola, M.D., Director, Life and Medicine Sciences Division, DOE
- John Pantaleo, M.S., Director, Isotope Programs, DOE
- Belinda Seto, Ph.D., Deputy Director, NIBIB, NIH
- George Mills, M.D., Director, Division of Medical Imaging & Hematology Products, Food and Drug Administration

A.6 SIXTH MEETING, FEBRUARY 19–20, 2007, WASHINGTON, D.C.

The objective of the sixth meeting was to gather information on developments at the DOE-Nuclear Energy's Isotope Programs. The following is the list of speakers for the open session:

- John Pantaleo, M.S., Director, Isotope Programs, DOE
- Darrell Fisher, Ph.D., Scientific Director, Pacific Northwest National Laboratory

Appendix B

Glossary and Acronyms

Accelerator: A machine used to accelerate charged particles to high energies to create radionuclides.

Agreement States: States to which the U.S. Nuclear Regulatory Commission (U.S. NRC) has transferred its regulatory authority. Transfer of U.S. NRC's authority to a state is an agreement that is signed by the governor of the state and the chairman of the commission.

Alpha particle: Subatomic matter consisting of two protons and two neutrons.

Antibody: A protein made by the immune system to detect and destroy foreign intruders, such as viruses and bacteria.

Antigen: Substances such as proteins that elicit an immune response.

Atherosclerosis: A cardiovascular disease in which fatty material builds up in the arteries.

Auger electron: The second electron that is ejected when emission of an initial electron from an atom causes an emission of a second electron.

Authorized user: The U.S. NRC regulates the use of radioactive material used in medicine by issuing licenses to medical facilities and users. Research using radioactive materials on human subjects may only be performed if the licensee has fulfilled the requirements outlined in 10 CFR Part 35, which include completing a minimum of 700 hours of training.

B-cells: Lymphocytes that are produced in the bone marrow, which play an important role in immune response.

Combinatorial library: Sets of compounds prepared using combinatorial chemistry, which allow scientists to access a wide range of substances and to search for compounds that bind to specific biological and non-biological targets.

Cyclotron: Circular accelerator.

Excitation function: The amount of radionuclide produced is dependent upon the energy of the particle with which the target is bombarded. The yield of the radioactive product versus the energy of the particle is called an excitation function.

Genomics: Describes molecular assessment of the entire genome.

Half-life: The length of time it takes for one-half of the radioactive material to decay by emitting radiation.

Hot atom chemistry: The study of the chemical reactions that occur between high-energy atoms or molecules.

Hypoxia: Shortage of oxygen or reduction in the concentration of oxygen in the environment.

Materials science: An interdisciplinary field comprising applied physics, chemistry, and engineering that studies the physical properties of matter and its applications.

Microfluidics: A multidisciplinary field that studies how fluids behave at microliter and nanoliter volumes and the design of systems in which small volumes of fluids will be used to provide automated sample processing, synthesis, separation, and measurements in devices commonly described by the term "lab-on-a-chip."

Minimal residual disease: Presence of residual malignant cells, even when few cancer cells can be detected by conventional means (i.e., at subclinical level).

Molecular imaging: Scientific discipline that studies new ways of imaging molecular events and biochemical reactions in a living organism using labeled tracers with high molecular specificity.

Monoclonal antibody: Antibodies that are identical and produced by one type of immune cell.

Nanotechnology: Broad scientific field that creates and uses materials and devices on the nanoscale (i.e., 10^{-9}).

Neurotransmitters: Chemicals that relay signals between the brain and other cells, for example, dopamine and serotonin.

Personalized medicine: Tailoring of strategies to detect, treat, and prevent disease based on an individual's genetic profile.

Pharmacodynamics: A branch of pharmacology that studies what a drug does to the body.

Pharmacokinetics: A branch of pharmacology that studies what the body does to the drug (i.e., how it is absorbed, distributed, metabolized, and excreted).

Positron: An elementary particle of antimatter that undergoes mutual annihilation with a nearby electron, which produces two gamma rays traveling in opposite directions.

Proteomics: Comprehensive analysis of the proteins found in cells and tissues.

Radionuclide: An atom with an unstable nucleus that emits gamma-rays, x-ray photons, or positrons, and also known as a radioisotope.

Radiopharmaceutical: Radioactive drug composed of a radionuclide and a pharmaceutical that is used for diagnosis or therapy.

Refractory disease: A condition that is unresponsive to treatment.

Scintillator: A substance that absorbs high-energy charged-particle radiation and then releases this energy through fluorescence.

Sensitivity: Percentage of radioactive decays that are detected by an imaging instrument.

Specific activity: Amount of radioactivity of a specific radionuclide or labeled compound divided by the mass of the radionuclide or labeled compound to which it has been incorporated.

Stage: A method of classifying patients by how far a disease has progressed.

Systems biology: A discipline that models the interactions within a biological system and studies how these interactions give rise to the function and behavior of that system.

Target: An element or chemical compound that is irradiated in an accelerator or reactor to produce a radionuclide.

Targeted radionuclide therapy: A form of treatment that delivers therapeutic doses of radiation to malignant tumors, for example, by administration of a radiolabeled molecule designed to seek out certain cells.

Targetry: Study of cyclotron target composition and structure to optimize the production of a desired nuclide from the "target" and minimize impurities made through nuclear reactions.

Time-of-flight: For each annihilation event the precise time that each of the coincident photons is detected is noted and the difference in arrival time is calculated.

Tracer: A measurable substance used to mimic, follow, or trace a chemical compound or element without perturbing the process.

ACRONYMS

ACRIN	American College of Radiology Imaging Network
AEC	Atomic Energy Commission
BERAC	Biological and Environmental Research Advisory Committee
BNL	Brookhaven National Laboratory
CEA	carcinoembryonic antigen
cGMP	current Good Manufacturing Practices
CMS	Centers for Medicare and Medicaid Services
CT	computed tomography
DOE	U.S. Department of Energy
DOE-NE	Department of Energy Office of Nuclear Energy
DOE-OBER	Department of Energy Office of Biological and Environmental Research
eIND	Exploratory Investigational New Drug
ERDA	Energy Research and Development Agency
FDA	U. S. Food and Drug Administration
FDG	2-deoxy-2-[^{18}F]fluoro-d-glucose (also called fluorodeoxyglucose)
GBM	glioblastoma multiforme
HIPAA	Health Insurance Portability and Accountability Act
IAEA	International Atomic Energy Agency
IND	Investigational New Drug
INL	Idaho National Laboratory
IRB	Institutional Review Board
LANL	Los Alamos National Laboratory
MIBG	meta-iodobenylguanidine
MRI	magnetic resonance imaging
MURR	Missouri University Research Reactor
NCI	National Cancer Institute
NEMA	National Electrical Manufacturers Association
NERAC	Nuclear Energy Research Advisory Committee
NHLBI	National Heart, Lung, and Blood Institute
NIBIB	National Institute of Biomedical Imaging and Bioengineering
NIDA	National Institute of Drug Abuse
NIH	National Institutes of Health
NIMH	National Institute of Mental Health
NINDS	National Institute of Neurological Disorders and Stroke
NRC	U.S. Nuclear Regulatory Commission
ORNL	Oak Ridge National Laboratory

PET   positron emission tomography
R&D   research and development
RIBBE   radiation-induced biological bystander effect
SPECT   single photon emission computed tomography
TRIUMF   Tri-University Meson Facility

Appendix C

Commercially Available Radiopharmaceuticals

Radiopharmaceutical	Trade Name	Primary Uses
Carbon-14 Urea	Pytest	Detection of H Pylori
Cobalt-57 cyanocobalamin	Rubratope	Schilling test
Chromium-51 sodium chromate	Chromitope (Bracco) Mallinckrodt Cr-51	Labeling red blood cells (RBC)
Fluorine-18-FDG		Positron emission tomography (PET) imaging
Gallium-67	Neoscan (GE) DuPont Ga-67 Mallinckrodt Ga-67	Soft-tissue tumor and inflammatory process imaging
Indium-111 chloride	Indiclor (Nycomed) Mallinckrodt In-111Cl	Labeling monoclonal antibodies and peptides (OncoScint & Octreoscan)
Indium-111 pentetate (DTPA)	Indium DTPA In-111	Imaging of cerebrospinal fluid kinetics
Indium-111 oxyquinoline (oxine)	Indium-111 oxine	Labeling leukocytes and platelets
Indium-111 Capromab pendetide	ProstaScint	Monoclonal antibody for imaging prostate cancer

Continued

Radiopharmaceutical	Trade Name	Primary Uses
Indium-111 pentetreotide	Octreoscan	Imaging neuroendocrine tumors
I-123 sodium iodide	Mallinckrodt Amersham	Thyroid imaging and uptake
I-125 iothalamate	Glofil	Measurement of glomerular filtration
I-125 human serum albumin (RISA)	Isojex	Plasma volume determinations
I-131sodium iodide	Iodotope (Bracco) CIS - I-131 Mallinckrodt I-131Soln Mallinckrodt I-131 Therapy Caps Mallinckrodt I-131 Diagnostic Caps	Thyroid uptake, imaging, and therapy
Tositumomab & Iodine I-131 Tositumomab	Bexxar	Treatment of non-Hodgkin's lymphoma
I-131 iodomethylnorcholesterol (NP-59)	(University of Michigan)	Adrenal imaging
I-131 metaiodobenzylguanidine (MIBG)	I-131 MIBG	Imaging pheochromocytomas and neuroblastomas
P-32 chromic phosphate	Phosphocol P32	Therapy for intracavitary malignancies
P-32 sodium phosphate		Therapy for polycythemia vera
Rubidium-82 (from Sr-82/Rb-82 generator)	Cardio-Gen-82	PET imaging
Samarium-153 Lexidronam (Sm-153 EDTMP)	Quadramet	Palliative treatment of bone pain of skeletal metastases
Strontium-89	Metastron	Palliative treatment of bone pain of skeletal metastases

Radiopharmaceutical	Trade Name	Primary Uses
Tc-99m pertechnetate Generators	DuPont Mallinckrodt DTE Mallinckrodt FM Amersham	Imaging thyroid, salivary glands, ectopic gastric mucosa, parathyroid glands, dacryocystography, cystography
Tc-99m Apcitide	AcuTect	Peptide imaging of deep vein thrombosis
Tc-99m bicisate (ECD)	Neurolite	Cerebral perfusion imaging
Tc-99m disofenin (DISIDA)	Hepatolite-CIS	Hepatobiliary imaging
Tc-99m exametazine (HMPAO)	Ceretec	Cerebral perfusion imaging
Tc-99m Gluceptate	Draximage Mallinckrodt	Renal imaging
Tc-99m human serum albumin (HSA)		Imaging cardiac chambers
Tc-99m macroaggregated albumin (MAA)	Pulmolite - CIS Macrotec (Bracco) Technescan MAA (Mallinckrodt) Draximage Amersham MAA	Pulmonary perfusion
Tc-99m Mebrofenin	Choletec	Hepatobiliary imaging
Tc-99m Medronate (MDP)	Bracco Osteolite - CIS Draximage Mallinckrodt Amersham	Bone imaging
Tc-99m Mertiatide	Technescan MAG3	Renal imaging
Tc-99m Oxidronate (HDP)	Mallinckrodt HDP	Bone imaging
Tc-99m Pentetate (DTPA)	Techneplex (Bracco) CIS-AN DTPA CIS-DTPA Draximage DTPA Mallinckrodt DTPA Nycomed DTPA	Renal imaging and function studies; Radioaerosol ventilation imaging

Continued

Radiopharmaceutical	Trade Name	Primary Uses
Tc-99m Pyrophosphate (PYP)	Phosphotec (Bracco) Pyrolite-CIS Pyro-CIS Technescan PYP Amersham PYP	Avid infarct imaging; in vivo RBC labeling
Tc-99m red blood cells	Ultratag	Imaging gastrointestinal (GI) bleeds, cardiac chambers
Tc-99m Sestamibi	Cardiolite Miraluma	Myocardial perfusion imaging Breast tumor imaging
Tc-99m Succimer (DMSA)	Amersham DMSA	Renal imaging
Tc-99m Sulfur Colloid (SC)	CIS-Sulfur Colloid Nycomed - SC	Imaging liver/spleen, gastric emptying, GI bleeds
Tc-99m Tetrofosmin	Myoview	Myocardial perfusion imaging
Thallium-201	DuPont Mallinckrodt Amersham	Myocardial perfusion imaging; Parathyroid and tumor imaging
Y-90 Ibitumomab Tiuxetan	Zevalin	non-Hodgkin's lymphoma
Xenon-133	DuPont Xenon Mallinckrodt Xenon Amersham Xenon	Pulmonary ventilation imaging
Interventional Agents	Trade Name	Use in nuclear medicine
ACD solution (anticoagulant acid Acitrate dextrose)	ACD Solution Modified	Anticoagulant used in blood labeling
Adenosine	Adenoscan	Pharmacologic stress
Ascorbic acid	Ascorbic acid	RBC labeling and HDP preparation
I.V. Dipyridamole	I.V. Persantine	Pharmacologic stress
Sincalide	Kinevac	Gallbladder ejection fraction studies

SOURCE: University of Arkansas for Medical Sciences (http://nuclearpharmacy.uams.edu/resources/PackageInserts.asp).

Appendix D

Biographical Sketches Of Committee Members

Hedvig Hricak, *Chair* (M.D., University of Zagreb; Ph.D., oncology, Karolinska Institute), is chairman of the Department of Radiology at Memorial Sloan-Kettering Cancer Center. Her expertise is in diagnostic radiology, particularly as it relates to imaging of genitourinary cancers. Her research studies use a variety of imaging methods including ultrasound, computed tomography, magnetic resonance imaging, and magnetic resonance imaging spectroscopy with the aim of improving cancer detecion, treatment planning, and follow-up. She was elected to the Institute of Medicine (IOM) in 2002. She received the Marie Curie Award from the Society of Women in Radiology in 2002 and the gold medal from the International Society for Magnetic Resonance in Medicine in 2003. She serves on the National Cancer Institute's Board of Scientific Advisors, on the Board of Directors of the Radiological Society of North America, and on the IOM's Committee on Cancer and Cancer Biology. She is an honorary member of the German Radiological Society, the British Institute of Radiology, and the Croatian Academy of Science and Art, and has an honorary doctorate in medicine from the Ludwig Maximilian University of Munich.

S. James Adelstein (M.D., Harvard Medical School; Ph.D., biophysics, Massachusetts Institute of Technology) is the Paul C. Cabot Distinguished Professor of Medical Biophysics at Harvard Medical School and a nuclear medicine specialist. His research interests are focused on the radiation biology and biophysics of internal emitters and the experimental treatment of cancer using radionuclides. He was elected to the Institute of Medicine in 1985. Dr. Adelstein is the vice-chair of the National Academies' Nuclear and Radiation Studies Board, was chair of the Board on Radiation Effects Research from 2002 to 2005 and has served on numerous National Research Council and IOM committees.

Peter S. Conti (M.D., Cornell University; Ph.D., biophysics, Cornell University) is professor of radiology, pharmacy, and biomedical engineering at the University of Southern California (USC), as well as director of the USC Positron Imaging Science Center and Clinic. He is board certified in nuclear medicine and diagnostic radiology, and his expertise is in the clinical use of positron emission tomography in the diagnosis, staging, and treatment of cancer. In addition, he is interested in the development of new radiolabeled imaging agents. He was the recipient of the Young Investigator Award by the American Society of Clinical Oncology and the postdoctoral award by Johns Hopkins Medical Institute in 1990. He is past president of the Society of Nuclear Medicine.

Joanna Fowler (Ph.D., chemistry, University of Colorado) is a senior chemist at Brookhaven National Laboratory and director of the Brookhaven PET Program. She has had a long-term interest in radiotracer synthesis with positron emitters and new applications of radiotracers in neuroscience. She was elected to the National Academy of Sciences (NAS) in 2003. She is the recipient of the Garvan-Olin Award and the Glen T. Seaborg Award from the American Chemical Society, the Paul Aebersold Award from the Society of Nuclear Medicine, and the E. O. Lawrence Award from the Department of Energy. She served on the NAS Panel on Benchmarking the Research Competitiveness of the U.S. in Chemistry and has served on the Committee on Nuclear and Radiochemistry and on the Board on Chemical Sciences and Technology.

Joe Gray (Ph.D., physics, Kansas State University) holds appointments as associate laboratory director for Life and Environmental Science at the Lawrence Berkeley National Laboratory (LBNL), director of the Division of Life Sciences at LBNL, and adjunct professor of laboratory medicine and radiation oncology at the University of California at San Francisco (UCSF). He also is program leader for breast oncology in the UCSF Comprehensive Cancer Center and is a member of UCSF's Program in Biological and Medical Informatics and the Graduate Group in Biophysics. His research interests include the development of analytic techniques in the study of cancer, and his current work focuses on the use of systems approaches to develop strategies to predict individual responses to agents that target signaling pathways regulating proliferation and/or apoptosis. Major awards include the E.O Lawrence Award from the Department of Energy, the Curt Stern Award from the American Society for Human Genetics, and the Leadership Award from the National Cancer Institute (NCI) Specialized Programs of Research Excellence. He has also served on the Science Council of the Radiation Effects Research Foundation and currently serves on the Board of Scientific Advisors for NCI.

Lin-wen Hu (Ph.D., nuclear engineering, Massachusetts Institute of Technology) is the associate director for research development and utilization at the Massachusetts Institute of Technology's Nuclear Reactor Laboratory (NRL). She directs NRL's research, irradiation services, and outreach activities and is responsible for the development, design, and safety reviews of major reactor experiments. In addition, she supervises NRL's radiochemistry laboratory, which specializes in trace elements analysis in biological samples. Her areas of expertise include research reactor applications and instrumental neutron activation for medical and environmental research. She has served as chair of the American Nuclear Society's isotopes and radiation division, which is devoted to applying nuclear engineering technologies related to isotopes and radiation in scientific research and medicine and industry.

Joel Karp (Ph.D., physics, Massachusetts Institute of Technology) is professor of radiology, the chief of the Physics and Instrumentation Research Section in the Department of Radiology, and director of the Department of Radiology PET Center at the University of Pennsylvania. His research interests focus on positron emission tomography (PET) instrumentation design, which includes development of scintillation detectors, data correction techniques, 3-dimensional image reconstruction algorithms, and evaluation of imaging performance for human and animal imaging studies. He has chaired the Institute of Electrical and Electronic Engineers (IEEE) Nuclear Medical and Imaging Sciences Council, and the Society of Nuclear Medicine PET Standards Committee. In addition, he is currently senior editor of *IEEE Transactions on Nuclear Science—Nuclear Medical Imaging Sciences.*

Thomas Lewellen (Ph.D., experimental nuclear physics, University of Washington) is professor of radiology, adjunct professor of electrical engineering, and director of physics and instrumentation development in nuclear medicine at the University of Washington. His research interests include the development of small animal PET systems and improving imaging capabilities for single photon emission computed tomography, PET, and PET/CT scanners for clinical use. He is a senior member of the Institute of Electrical and Electronic Engineers and the recipient of the Bronze Medal Award for Physics from the Society of Nuclear Medicine, the Innovative Technology Award from National Aeronautics and Space Administration, and the Distinguished Scientist Award from the Western Regional Society of Nuclear Medicine.

Roger Macklis (M.D., Harvard Medical School) is professor of medicine at the Cleveland Clinic Lerner College of Medicine. His expertise is in radiation oncology, and his major research interests include biologically targeted radiopharmaceutical therapy, pediatric radiation oncology, and clinical research in breast cancer, lymphomas, and brain tumor radiotherapy. He has received the Young Investigator Award from the American Society of Clinical Oncology, Resident Research Award from the American Society for Therapeutic Radiology and Oncology, and the Junior Faculty Research Award from the American Cancer Society, among other honors. He has served as radiation oncology representative for the National Wilms' Tumor Study Group and currently serves as an examiner for the American Board of Radiology.

C. Douglas Maynard (M.D., Wake Forest University School of Medicine) is the former chairman of the Radiology Department at Wake Forest University School of Medicine and is currently professor emeritus of radiology. His expertise is in diagnostic radiology (nuclear medicine), with a special interest in the applications of engineering to medical imaging. In this capacity, he helped establish the National Institute of Biomedical Imaging and Bioengineering at the National Institutes of Health. He has also served as past president of the Academy of Radiology Research, the Radiological Society of North America, the American Board of Radiology, and the Society of Nuclear Medicine. In addition, he was awarded the Medallion of Merit, the highest honor bestowed from Wake Forest University, in 2002.

Thomas Ruth (Ph.D., nuclear spectroscopy, Clark University) is director of the PET Program at the University of British Columbia. He is a leader in the production and application of radioisotopes for research in the physical and biological sciences. His efforts at establishing PET as a quantitative tool for in vivo biochemistry has been recognized by the Canadian Nuclear Medicine Society's highest award of Meritorious Status. He has served on a multitude of committees, including the National Research Council's Committee on Medical Isotope Production.

Heinrich Schelbert (M.D., University of Würzburg; Ph.D., biology, University of Würzburg) is the George V. Taplin Professor at the David Geffen School of Medicine of the University of California at Los Angeles. He is also an attending of the clinical nuclear medicine service. His research interests focus on the development and validation of noninvasive radionuclide imaging techniques for the study of cardiovascular function. He has received the Distinguished Scientific Achievement Award from the American Heart Association, the Distinguished Clinical Scientist Award from the Academy of Molecular Imaging, and is a two-time recipient of the Georg von Hevesy Prize by the World Federation of Nuclear Medicine and Biology. In addition, he is currently the editor-in-chief of the *Journal of Nuclear Medicine.*

Gustav von Schulthess (M.D., Harvard Medical School; Ph.D., physics, Massachusetts Institute of Technology) is professor of nuclear medicine at the University Hospital of Zurich and was previously a visiting professor in the Department of Radiology at Stanford University. His research interests include the clinical applicability of combined positron emission tomography (PET) and computed tomography (CT), or PET/CT, particularly as it relates to tumor imaging. He has received the Seroussi Memorial Award and a research award from the Swiss Radiological Society.

Michael R. Zalutsky (Ph.D., nuclear chemistry, Washington University) is professor of radiology, professor of biomedical engineering, and associate professor of pathology at Duke University Medical Center. His expertise is in radiology, particularly as it relates to antibody therapy. His primary research interest is developing novel radioactive compounds for improving the diagnosis and treatment of cancer. Honors he has received include the Berson-Yalow Award from the Society of Nuclear Medicine in 2005, the MERIT (Method to Extend Research in Time) Award from the National Cancer Institute, and the Wilhelm Manchot Visiting Professorship at Technische Universität Munich. He has served on the National Institutes of Health's special study sections, such as in radiotherapeutic applications, radiolabeled antibodies for breast cancer, and radiation oncology applications, and is a reviewer for proposals on nuclear medicine for the Department of Energy.

3/21/08